AV HEALTH

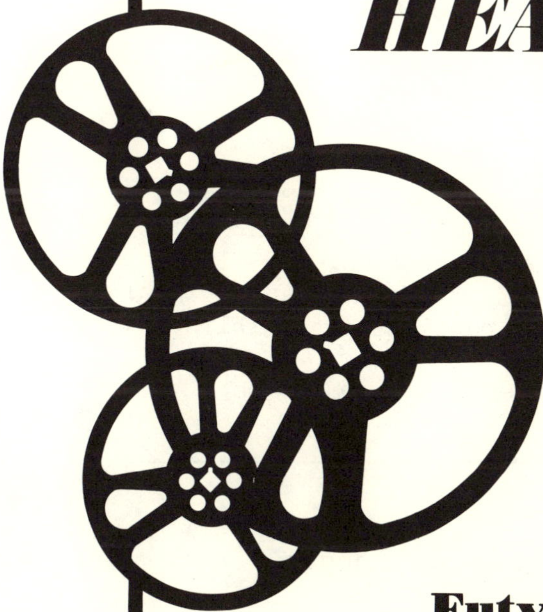

Current Publications of The United States Government

by

Eutychia G. Londos

The Scarecrow Press • Metuchen, N.J., & London • 1982

Cover Design: Eutychia G. Londos

Graphics: Janice Rajecki

Library of Congress Cataloging in Publication Data

Londos, Eutychia G.
  AV health.

  Includes indexes.
  1. Health--Audio-visual aids--Catalogs. 2. Health education--Audio-visual aids--Catalogs. 3. United States--Government publications--Catalogs. I. Title. II. Title: A.V. health. [DNLM: 1. Health--Audiovisual aids--Catalogs. 2. Government publications--Bibliography. ZWA 18 L847a]
RA440.3.U5L66 1982   016.3621   82-10366
ISBN 0-8108-1571-0

Copyright © 1982 by Eutychia G. Londos

Manufactured in the United States of America

DEDICATED

to the nation of immigrants,
to America

Contents

ACKNOWLEDGEMENTS	i
FOREWORD	iii
INTRODUCTION	vii
PLATES	xv
PUBLICATIONS	1
SPECIAL ITEMS	127
AGENCIES	141
TITLE INDEX	153
SUBJECT INDEX	159

Acknowledgements

With rare exceptions, this is not a book done from experience alone. My own experience with health sciences audiovisuals encompasses only the last nine or ten years of audiovisuals' one hundred-year reign, and if I had attempted to trust only my own expereince, I could have hardly brought together this "reservoir" of knowledge and information that the United States Government has provided the health scientist, the public, and the world. He who attempts a book of this type is one of the most indebted of men. So many individuals contributed and assisted in so many known and unknown ways. All that can be said is to humbly acknowledge their generous assistance. Among those are the personnel employed in the following agencies of the United States Government:

Academy of the Health Sciences United States Army (AHSUSA); Administration on Aging; Department of Agriculture; Alcohol, Drug Abuse, and Mental Health Administration; Bureau of Alcohol, Tobacco, and Firearms; Animal and Plant Health Inspection; Armed Forces Institute of Pathology; Army Audiovisual Center; Army Fifth Headquarters; Department of the Army Headquarters; Army Training Support Center; Audiovisual Archives Division of the National Archives and Records Service; Center for Disease Control; Civil Aeronautics Board; Department of Commerce; Community Services Administration; Office of Consumer Affairs; Consumer Education and Awareness; Consumer Inquiries; Consumer Product Safety Commission; Department of Defense; Drug Enforcement Administration; Bureau of Drugs; Bureau of Education for the Handicapped; Department of Energy; Energy Resources and Development Administration; Environmental Protection Agency; Federal Aviation Administration; Federal Emergency Management Agency; Federal Highway Administration; Federal Maritime Commission; Food and Drug Administration; Food and Nutrition Information and Educational Materials Center; Food and Nutrition Service; Food Safety and Quality Service; Forest Service of Eastern and Pacific Northwest Regions; Department of Health and Human Service; Bureau of Health Manpower; Health Resources Administration; Health Services Administration; Department of Housing and Urban Development; Bureau of Indian Affairs; ICRDB Program (International Cancer Research Data Bank); Interdepartmental Committee on Visual and Auditory Materials for Distribution Abroad; Department of the Interior; International Communication Agency; International Development Cooperation Agency (Agency for International Development); Department of Justice; Department of Labor; Law Enforcement Assistance Administration; Library of Congress; Minnesota Department of Natural Resources; Mine Safety and Health Administration; National Aeronautics and Space Administration; National Audiovisual Center; National Bureau of Standards; National Cancer Institute; National Center on Child Abuse and Neglect;

National Clearinghouse for Drug Abuse Information; National Endowment of the Humanities; National Foundation of the Arts and the Humanities; National Heart, Lung, and Blood Institute; National High Blood Pressure Education Program; National Highway and Safety Administration; National Industrial Council—Office of Field Operations—Office of Energy Programs—U.S. Department of Domestic and International Business Administration; National Institute of Arthritis, Metabolism, and Digestive Diseases; National Institute of Child Health and Human Development; National Institute of Drug Abuse Resource Center; National Institute of Education; National Institute for Environmental Sciences; National Institutes of Health; National Institute of Mental Health; National Institute of Neurological, Communicable Disorders, and Stroke; National Institute of Occupational Safety and Health; National Library of Medicine; National Medical Audiovisual Center; National Oceanic and Atmospheric Administration; National Safety Council; National Science Foundation; National Technical Information Service; Naval Health Sciences Education and Training Command; Department of the Navy; Nuclear Regulatory Commission; Office of Communications and Public Affairs; Office of Education; Office of Human Development; Office of Personnel Management; President's Committee on Mental Retardation; President's Committee on Physical Fitness and Sports; Bureau of Prisons; Public Health Service; Bureau of Radiological Health; Rehabilitation Services Administration; Smithsonian Institution; Social Rehabilitation Service; Superintendent of Documents; Veterans Administration; Veterans Administration Dental Training Center; Veterans Administration Medicine and Surgery Department; U.S. Coast Guard; U.S. Fish and Wildlife Service; and West Point of U.S. Military Academy.

In the matter of retrieving publications—I am indebted to the staff of: Government Documents Department of the University of Illinois at Chicago Circle; the Government Publications Department of the Chicago Public Library; and the Reference Department of the Regenstein Library of the University of Chicago who spent hours searching through thousands of documents and loaned me materials I might otherwise have missed altogether.

And a final, special thanks to Catherine Nelson for the final preparation of the manuscript.

E.G.L.

Foreword

The recent completed report of the National Commission on Libraries and Information Sciences, *Problems in Bibliographic Access to Non-Print Materials,* stated that

> effective success of audiovisual productions cannot be achieved without first establishing control.

One of those concerned with the dissemination of this type of materials is the United States Government. Its agencies have been publishing catalogs and indexes since the turn of the century with the intent to make their productions available to the users not only in a single nation but also to the world. There are approximately 175 producing Government agencies, and approximately the same number of publications. One hundred and thirty of them include exclusively medical and allied health programs. Many of these publications have expanded their scope and include programs produced by non-U.S. Government agencies such as independent producers, associations, organizations, educational institutions, private business institutions, and governments around the world.

The process of retrieving and distributing the materials included in these publications becomes more complex as information continues to expand at a very rapid rate. Locating these materials becomes a difficult task for the user, as there is no single comprehensive listing of both the audiovisual materials or their sources. This book has two major purposes—to bring together in one volume uncoordinated pieces of information which accumulates in Government collections with the hope that these collections will become more accessible, and also, to serve as a stimulus to other health professionals interested in developing tools for better dissemination of audiovisual productions productions and publications of the United States Government.

SCOPE It organizes publications and their content methodologically for easy retrieval and dissemination of materials. Each publication, regardless of its title, contains health sciences audiovisuals for the professional as well as for the layperson, and therefore, should be examined individually.

> Example A. *A List of Audiovisual Materials Produced by the U.S. Government in History,* includes
> Aviation Medicine
> Chemical, psychological, and tactical air warfare

       Concentration camps—victims of medical experiments
       Food and medical assistance to civilians during wars
       Government programs on conservation, agriculture, and natural resources
       Hospitals overseas during wars, and Civil and Spanish wars
       Nursing—training
       Research on medical knowledge in the field of obstetrics

    Example B. *Documentary Film Classics,* includes
       Agriculture
       The Chicago Maternity Center
       Crimes against humanity
       Death
       Environmental sciences
       Hunger and poverty
       Irrigation
       Occupational health and preventive medicine
       Psychology
       Social issues
       Wars and their casualties

EDITIONS Publications included are current, but a few earlier editions, with highly specialized content and which are still available, are included for those involved in research and scientific comparisons. Many programs in those publications are scientifically sound and considered of historical value. For information on the availability of these materials, write to the National Audiovisual Center.

SUBJECT CONTROL A comprehensive Subject Index is provided based on the National Library of Medicine's Medical Subject Headings *(MeSH),* and the Library of Congress *(LC).* Other terminology which appears in individual publications is translated into *MeSH* and *LC* and also included in the "Miscellaneous" section within the Subject Index.

    Example A. *Bionomics,* appears in the following subjects:
       1. biology
       2. bionomics (Miscellaneous)
       3. ecology
       4. environmental sciences

    Example B. *Terradynamics,* appears in the following subjects:
       1. energy
       2. engineering
       3. physics
       4. terradynamics (Miscellaneous)

  Because of the complex, diverse, and highly specialized content, some of the publications have been also indexed in the "Miscellaneous" section within the Subject Index listed under special subjects.

Example A.   CPR (Cardiopulmonary Resuscitation)
A List of Audiovisual Materials Produced by the U.S. Government for Emergency Medical Service
A List of Audiovisual Materials Produced by the U.S. Government—Spanish Soundtracks
Source Book of Educational Materials for Radiation Therapy

Example B.   "Walt Disney" Classic Health Series
A Guide to Audiovisual Aids for Spanish-Speaking Americans
Health: Selected List of Books that Have Appeared in Talking Book Topics and Braille Book Review
Health, 1980-81

In addition, the user might find in the same section items like cinematography (medical), Three Mile Island, baby sitters, disorientation, Fermi Laboratory—discovery of plutonium, and other health related and non-related topics.

ASTERISK (*)   An asterisk (*) identifies publications which are comprehensive in scope in that they include educational and instructional audiovisual programs classified under *MeSH* and *LC* subject headings which are constantly expanded.

ELEMENTS OF ENTRIES   Publications are listed alphabetically under title with complete bibliographic information. Each title is followed by: 1) type of media (format), 2) summary, giving number of entries, subjects—listed in alphabetical order, currency of materials, level of audience (when available), availability, producer(s), authors (when applicable), and award(s), 3) bibliographic information on entries, 4) special features (indexes, producers and distributors, TV clearance, 5) accompanying print material(s), 6) language if other than English, 7) country of origin, 8) miscellaneous information, 9) ordering information, and 10) price(s) of publications or free-loan information.

PRICES   Prices included are quoted as they appear in various indexes at the time of publication of this book. The Subject Bibliography MOTION PICTURES, FILMS, AND AUDIOVISUAL INFORMATION, published by the U.S. Government Printing Office (included in this book), indicates that prices are subject to change without prior notice.

INQUIRIES   This book was made possible by the interest of the U.S. Government agencies to make their audiovisual productions and publications available by supplying the author with complimentary copies of their publications and also directing inquiries to the appropriate source. To obtain copies of individual publications, send requests to perspective publishing agencies listed in this book. In addition, all Government agencies dealing with audiovisuals are listed in the *Directory of U.S. Audiovisual Personnel*, published by the National Audiovisual Center, which serves as Clearinghouse of the Government audiovisuals. Those seeking information on special subjects, should write to the National Audiovisual Center, National Archives and Records Service, General Services Administration, Washington, D.C. 20409.

Eutychia G. Londos

Introduction

Mankind has always tried to convey information to one another. The earliest known record of man's activities are depicted in drawings, characters, and symbols as an attempt to impart knowledge. European cave paintings revealed drawings of animals which man encountered and artifacts which he used. The hieroglyphics of Egypt and the characters of China paved the way to the sculptures of ancient Greece and the paintings of medieval Italy.

As mankind continued to learn through such writings and paintings, specific beliefs developed and became incorporated into an educational philosophy. John Amos Comenius (1592-1671) felt that learning could be enhanced by pictures. His "Orbus Pictus" or the "World Illustrated" was the first textbook to use pictures. It was used for nearly a century in Europe. Another belief developed in education which has persisted to the current time. Pestalozzi (1746-1827) developed the theory that the senses of sight and touch needed to be strengthened in order to increase learning. This concept was furthered by Froebal (1782-1852) who insisted on the use of visual aids in his kindergarten.[1]

From that time to the present, learning has been encouraged with a variety of visual aids such as blackboard and textbook drawings, maps, charts, and photographs. The use of the latter became widespread after 1822 when Niepce, a Frenchman, developed a way to record a photograph permanently. Many other inventions, including the development of a sensitized medium to record photographs and the use of specific equipment for taking and showing pictures, led to the use of the stereoscope and the lantern slide as instructional aids. Eventually, the use of a series of pictures presented in rapid succession made the pictures appear as if they were moving. Thus the "motion picture" industry was born.

In 1892, Dr. Sellers of Philadelphia patented the Kinematoscope which recorded the use of real people in continuing action. In 1892, Eadweard Muybridge, an Englishman who was engaged in the official duties as a photographer of the U.S. Government for the Pacific Coast, analyzed the movement of objects, including horses running at the racetrack. For twenty years he had worked on the scientific concept of movement until he developed the Zoopraxoscope, a machine which projected moving pictures onto a screen to enable many people to visualise the movement. Dr. Marey, a French scientist, was concerned with the use of motion pictures to enhance man's knowledge of the sciences. He and Muybridge's work involved recording scientific information.[2]

This scientific invention fascinated the U.S. Government personnel. A young clerk working for the United States Treasury in Washington, D.C., Francis Jenkins, studied Edison's Kinetoscope, Anschutz's Tachyscope, and Muybridge's work. The goal of these men was to project life-size motion pictures on a screen. As early as 1890, Jenkins also began trying to develop a similar machine. He experimented using a revolving lens system (PLATE I), but apparently his projector did not operate efficiently. With persistence he perfected the system and his first public performance received newspaper attention on June 6, 1894, in Richmond, Indiana.[3]

At the Chicago's World's Fair in 1892, Muybridge exhibited his machine, the Zoopraxoscope,[4] and at the same time, Edison exhibited his Kinetograph, the first motion picture to use film . Other inventors added to the refinement of motion pictures and in 1896, New Yorkers had the opportunity to see the first motion picture show when moving pictures were viewed on a theater screen. Of course, it was not until the 1920s that sound was added to sight to create the "talkies." However, it was both the emergence of audiovisual materials as significant tools of instruction and sources of information, and the beginning of the motion picture industry.

Among the first to utilize the great invention of motion pictures was the United States Government. In 1907, the United States Reclamation Service exhibited at the Jamestown Exposition a film concerning its work of reclaiming arid lands.[5] In 1909, at the Alaskan-Yukon-Pacific Exposition, Joseph Abel, a photographer in the Bureau of Agriculture, filmed a livestock show. The Bureau was the first to use both motion picture and animation in a film studying wheat rust.[6]

Soon other films were made and used to educate students in agriculture. In 1912, the Office of Motion Picture Service was established in the Department. This Office was to coordinate the motion picture activities of all seventeen bureaus within the Department. During World War I, a Committee of Public Information was established to produce and distribute instructional and inspirational pictures. American-made films were sent to Russia at the end of the war to teach rural people about the various aspects of life such as agricultural methods and veterinary medicine.[7]

The Children's Bureau of the Department of Labor, with professional assistance from the infant specialist, Dr. Roger Dennet, produced many films among them a series on mothercraft, which were screened in commercial theaters during the 1914 "Baby Week" in New York.[8] By 1920, other agencies within the Department also produced films concerned with a variety of topics such as problems of unemployment, health, safety, and industrial hygiene. The Children's Bureau continued producing health sciences films, and with the cooperation of the industry and well known Hollywood personalities, audiovisuals produced during and immediately after World War II by the Bureau were deposited at the UNICEF (United Nations International Children's Emergency Fund) library where thousands of people all over the world viewed them. An example of these films is the "Assignment Children," an account of Danny Kaye's world tour on behalf of UNICEF, which shows prevention and cure of yaws, tuberculosis, malaria, and other diseases of children around the world. Films concerning children's health produced by the U.S. Government between 1945-1956 are on polio in Greece, leprosy in Africa, and rheumatic fever and child abuse in America, which were made in the United States for a world-wide distribution.[9] By 1950, The Children's Bureau had produced nearly 480 films for public use and included new topics such as child development and day care centers for working mothers.[10] Many of these productions (films, filmstrips, still photographs) are still available through UNICEF and WHO (World Health Organization) libraries.[11]

The United States National Advisory Committee for Aeronautics began to make films in 1915 with the help of the Wright Brothers. During World War II, this department conducted studies on the effects of gravity, low temperatures, and low pressure on human subjects. The National Aeronautics and Space Administration (NASA) was organized in 1958 and has continued producing films as space research continues.[12]

The United States Army was the first military department to produce motion pictures. During World War I, the Medical Department of the Army made educational films to train personnel. In 1918, a specific Army Group Museum Unit was organized to film medical activities. The Unit was sent overseas where it visited practically every medical hospital on the "Western Front" and photographed all aspects of war and its effects on personnel. These photographs were forwarded to the United States and were used by medical students as if they had been "over there."[13] After the War, Army personnel was deeply involved in both photography and scientific camera inventions. One of these inventions was the automatic microphotographic camera designed in 1933 by Dr. R.H. Dreager, a Lieutenant Officer of the Medical Corps, U.S. Army (PLATE II). This invention made the U.S. Army also the first to duplicate audiovisual works, as well as print materials, and thousands of medical programs were placed in libraries for public use in the United States and abroad.[14] It was followed by the United States Public Health Service most comprehensive 35mm photographic apparatus installations invented by Earle and Crisp noted for their work in carcinogens.[15]

Wartime needs stimulated and accelerated the development of the factual film in many fields. The Public Health Service's films depicted health problems in crowded city streets, immigrant conditions at Ellis Island, and unsanitary conditions of food. These films were shown throughout the country in order to teach the public how to combat communicable diseases and to improve personal hygiene.[16] As well as the production of films for the public, films were also made for specialized audiences such as medical personnel. The Public Health Service Act of July 1944 extended the services and research of the agency by consolidating and revising all existing legislation relating to public health service. This was the beginning of large scale film production in all aspects of health services.

The Immigration and Naturalization Service in the 1920s produced a variety of films to help new citizens deal with cultural problems. The Department of the Interior films taught the public about irrigation and water purification. One of the seventeen federal government agencies producing motion pictures by 1920 was the Radio and Visual Section of the Office of Education, then a part of the Department of the Interior. This agency produced the first driver training film.[17] In the 1930s, the United States National Emergency Council, the Tennessee Valley Authority, the Works Progress Administration, and numerous other agencies were all producing motion pictures dealing with their respective fields. Following World War II, the films produced by the wartime departments were transferred to the Office of Education for dissemination.[18]

Because of the vast number of motion pictures being produced by Government agencies as well as private industries, the United States Congress in 1926 proposed a federal motion picture committee to regulate film activities and to protect the viewer from inaccurate media content. The Committee, after appraising such educational films, found that they were produced on a highly professional level.[19]

Although the increasing number of Government agencies continued to produce films concerning their respective fields, in 1942 the Army recognized the need to train millions of men and women in medical survival techniques. In 1944, the Navy developed slides and filmstrips concerning neurotic and psychotic conditions which were used by medical personnel for many years. Within the years 1941-1945, the Armed Forces produced more than six times the number of motion pictures for educational use than had ever been produced before.[20] Other agencies involved in film-making were the Department of Commerce, National Youth Administration of the Federal Security Administration, the Armed Forces Institute of Pathology, and the Academy of the Health Sciences United States Army. In 1949, the National Mental Health Film Board and the Cancer Institute were formed and also produced films representing their respective concerns.

When World War II ended, the Armed Forces, the largest audiovisual producer, ceased its grand scale production activities, and in the 1950s, the Government was more concerned with distribution and research than with production. But with the passage of the 1958 National Defense Education Act (Title VII), studies were conducted to see what effect audiovisuals had on learning. As a result, during the 60s, the rate of production soared, and it is difficult to count the thousands of health sciences audiovisuals made over the last two decades.[21] And although since World War II certain Government agencies were terminated or incorporated into others, the establishment of new departments began, many of them involved in audiovisual production. However, as each department continued to produce films, some agencies worked together to produce documentaries. The President's Committee on "Employment of the Handicapped," for example, won the Award for Creative Excellence in Documentary category at the 1977 United States Industrial Film Festival.[22]

The expansion of scientific knowledge has caused the proliferation of audiovisual materials. This expansion has also brought with it, in turn, difficulties of bibliographic control. From the first "moving picture" to the complex films from outer space, the need to document scientific phenomena, preserve them, and disseminate them to those involved in the health sciences around the world has been of importance. As early as 1903, a strong plea was made in Madrid, Spain, for preservation, bibliographic control, and dissemination by many professional and technical people who were dealing with their development and use. They proposed the creation of International Archives and Libraries.[23] In 1952, the Centre International Du Film Medical in Paris, France, listed 8,000 medical film titles which had been produced around the world.[24]

In the United States, the Government also was concerned with the dissemination of such information. In 1910, president Taft himself took actual participation in the distribution of the film "Life of the Fly," which dealt with sanitation problems. This was one of the first films with a health message to be shown to the public. In 1912, the president financed a film group to produce the first industrial hygiene motion picture, which was viewed by hundreds of people and served as a campaign to promote workers' health and safety.[25] In 1930, the U.S. Government created the Commission on Implications of Armed Services Education Program which explored the use of audiovisuals with the view to their adaptability to the American education system. Thousands of educators, artists, medical experts, and advertisers were involved in the production and dissemination of the audiovisual materials.[26] Since then, audiovisual publications listing films available to the public were published by the Government irregularly, bringing together both government and non-government productions of audiovisuals. But this task is always difficult. The creation of new agencies within the Federal Government as well as old agencies producing audiovisuals created a Herculean task of documentation. In 1912, the Department of Agriculture attempted to spread information about its educational films by various means such as bulletins, press, radio and exhibitions. In 1920, the Department's Motion Pictures Service published its first catalog, as an annual publication. By 1932, comprehensive catalogs listing hundreds of subjects were published.[27] The Office of Education distributed lists of films, exhibits, slides, and maps to science teachers in 1937. In 1938, the United States Film Service of the Division of the National Emergency Council prepared the first comprehensive catalog entitled THE DIRECTORY OF UNITED STATES GOVERNMENT FILMS.[28] The first catalog of medical and biological films was issued in 1946.

The pioneer work for bibliographic control and dissemination of such materials produced by both government and independent agencies and make them available to potential users not only in a single nation but also to the world was initiated by the U.S. Library of Congress. Under the Act of 1903, the Library of Congress became the depository and disseminating center of all audiovisual materials produced by the government, but because of financial problems, this project was abandoned. However, in 1949, the Library did publish its first catalog, GUIDE TO U.S. GOVERNMENT MOTION PICTURES, which was intended to be an annual publication.[29] But the Motion Picture Division was liquidated under the 1948 Legislative Branch Appropriations Act. Finally, in 1952, the Library broadened the activities of bibliographic control and dissemination of audiovisuals and began publishing standard reference cards for medical motion pictures and filmstrips produced by both government agencies and commercial producers released in the United States and Canada.[30]

In 1975, the National Library of Medicine (NLM), in addition to comprehensive catalogs published by the library which include health sciences audiovisual materials pro-

duced nationally and internationally,[31] created the computerized system called the AVLINE-Audiovisual On-Line which includes audiovisuals produced by both government and independent producers. It was hoped that by steady expansion the database would consist of 10,000 health science entries by 1982.[32]

In 1977, the government created the National Audiovisual Center (NAC) under the aegis of the National Archives and Records Service of the General Services Administration to serve as the Central Clearinghouse for all audiovisual materials produced by the 175 government producing agencies. The Center's catalog, REFERENCE OF AUDIOVISUAL MATERIALS PRODUCED BY THE UNITED STATES GOVERNMENT and its Special Subject Issues, include approximately 13,000 entries, many of which are in the health sciences area.[33]

During the last two decades, government audiovisual publications in the health sciences have been proliferating to keep up with the rapid production of materials produced not only by the U.S. Government agencies, but also by commercial and independent producers, professional associations, medical schools and universities from around the world. Today, there are more than 200 audiovisual catalogs published by the U.S. Government. Approximately 130 of them list only health science materials produced by their perspective agency, while others list both government and non-government productions which include a variety of subjects. Newer publications appear which include materials either converted to the new audiovisual technology or available in the original format. The U.S. Government sporadically publishes medical catalogs of various topics, also.[34]

Although the Government has produced numerous films to aid education and research of medical and scientific conditions, the public is often unaware that most of such films are free of charge in the United States and abroad. This book has been compiled with the knowledge that with the proliferation of audiovisual topics and the expansion of Government agencies many educators and health care personnel are not aware of such a source of learning.

The author has given us a comprehensive account of the state-of-the art of the United States Government Audiovisual Publications in the Health Sciences, which have been produced to convey information to others. The earliest known record of man's activities was to import knowledge to others. This book is an initial attempt to continue that endeavor.

Faith M. Jones, Ed. D.

BIBLIOGRAPHY

[1] Ellis, Don Carlos, and Thornborough, Laura. Motion Pictures in Education. New York, Thomas Y. Crowell Company, 1923. p. 1-3.

[2] Muybridge, E. Letter to the Editor. La Nature, February 17, 1879.

[3] Jenkins, Charles Francis. Vision by Radio, Radio Photographs, Radio Photography by C. Francis Jenkins... [Washington, D.C., Capital Press], inc. [1925]. 23 p.

[4] Muybridge, Eadweard. Descriptive Zoopraxography on the Science of Animal Locomotion Made Popular, by Eadweard Muybridge.... Published as a Memento of a Series of Lectures Given by the Author

Under the Auspices of the United States Government, Bureau of Education, at the World's Columbia Exposition, in Zoopraxographical Hall, 1893. [Philadelphia] University of Pennsylvania, [Chicago, the Lakeside Press] 1893. p. i, xi, 44, 34, 14.

Annual Report Board of Regents of the Smithsonian Institution, for the year ending June 30, 1901. Washington, U.S. Government Printing Office. 1902. p. 317-334.

[5] Jamestown Exposition 1907... Official Guide of the Jamestown centennial exposition held at Sewell's Point on Hampton Roads, near Norfolk, Va., April 26 to November 30, 1907. Copl. by W.H. Bright, Norfolk, Va., A. Hess, c1907. p. 112.

[6] Seattle, Alaska-Yukon-Pacific Exposition, 1909. Prize list, rules and regulations (preliminary). Department of live-stock. [Seattle, Challenge Press, 1909]. p. 121.

[7] Ellis, op, cit., p. 17-19; 113.

[8] Dench, Ernest A. Motion Picture Education, by Ernest A. Dench. Cincinnati. The Standards Publishing Company, [1916]. p. 182-183.

[9] Selected Films on Child Life. Children's Bureau, U.S. Department of Health, Education, and Welfare, 1962. 114 p. [Children's Bureau Publication No. 376].

[10] International Index of Films and Film Strips on the Health and Welfare of Children. United States Educational Scientific and Cultural Motion Pictures and Filmstrips Suitable and Available for Use Abroad. U.S. Commission for the United Nations Educational, Scientific, and Cultural Organization—Panel on Education Films 1950, Department of State (GPO State—130) Supplement 1951, 1952. 90 p. (U.S. Government productions covered 21 pages in various pagings).

[11] Motion Pictures. Med. Biol. Illus. 7:123, 1957.

[12] O'Hara, Frederic J. Bibliographic Essays on Government Documents and Diverse Matters. New York, Long Island University Palmer Graduate School, 1973. p. EX-X-1-4.

[13] Nichtenhauser, Adolf. A History of Motion Pictures in Medicine. Prepared for the Audio-Visual Training Section, Professional Training Division, Bureau of Medicine and Surgery, Department of the Army. 7 Vols. 2:150-180, [1951]. Available from the Naval Health Sciences Education and Training Command National Naval Medical Center, Bethesda, Md.

[14] Fussler, Herman H. Photographic Reproduction for Libraries: A Study of Administrative Problems. Chicago, University of Chicago Press, 1944. p. 140-153. "Several of this type of cameras made by various men in the 30's are described and illustrated by V.D. Tate in *"The Present Status of Equipment and Supplies for Microphotography," Journal of Documentary Reproduction,* I, No. 3 (Summer, 1938), 1-62. (Footnote p. 141).

[15] Earle, W.R., and Crisp, I.R. *Microcinematographic Equipment.* J. Nat. Cancer Inst. 1943, 4, 174. Private Communication, May 1953. From W.R. Earle, *Tissue Culture Section,* Department of Health, Education, and Welfare, U.S. Public Health Service, Bethesda, Md.

[16] Moving Picture World. 20:1250, 1914.

[17] Sprague, L.W. Motion Pictures in Public Health. Nation's Health. I:330, 1919.

[18] Hoban, Charles F., and Van Ormer, Edward B. Instructional Film Research (Rapid Mass Learning) 1918-

1950. Technical report No. SDC 269-7-19, the Instructional Film Research Program, Special Devices Center, Fort Washington, L.I., New York, 1951.

ANONYMOUS. Motion Picture Research Summarized. Journal of Medical Education. 28:63-67.

[19] U.S. Congress. Proposed Federal Motion Picture Commission. Hearings Report, Committee on Education House of Representatives. Sixty-Nine Congress, Frist Session on N.R. 4094 and N.R. 6233. Washington, U.S. Govt. Print. Off. 1926.

[20] Miles, John R., and Spain, Charles, R. Commission on Implications Armed Services Educational Programs. Audio-Visual Aids in the Armed Services. Washington, American Council on Education, 1947.

[21] Lumsdaine, Arthur A. Instruments and Media Instruction. Handbook of Research on Teaching. Chicago, Rand McNally, 1963. p. 583-682.

[22] U.S. Library of Congress. Division for the Blind and Physically Handicapped. Catalog of Caption Films for the Deaf/Catalog of Braille Book Review/Catalog of Talking Book/Catalog of Cassette Books. Library of Congress Media Services and Captioned Films, Bureau of Education for the Handicapped. Washington, D.C., Library of Congress.

[23] Donaldson, L. The Cinematograph and Natural Sciences. London, Ganes, 1912.

[24] CENTRE INTERNATIONAL DU DILM MEDICAL. 3 Rue de Siam, Paris XVI, France.

[25] ... House Fly Actors Make Their Debut on the Stage. Moving Picture World 6:375, 1910.

[26] Miles, John R., and Spain, Charles R., op. cit., p. 27-30.

[27] Koon, Cline. U.S. Bureau of Naval Personnel Training Manual. Basic United States Navy Manual as Educational Use of Film Strips and Instructional Motion Pictures. A Training Manual Prepared under the Supervision of the Bureau of Naval Personnel. Washington, U.S. Government Print. Off. 1942. p. 96-97.

[28] U.S. Film Service. Directory of U.S. Government Films 1938. National Emergency Council, Washington, D.C., 1938. 17 p.

[29] The Library of Congress as the National Bibliographic Center; Report of a Program Sponsored by the Association of Research Libraries, October 16, 1976. Washington, D.C., Association of Research Libraries, 1976. p. 56.

[30] Londos, Eutychia G. Compendium of Current Source Materials for Drugs. Metuchen, N.J., The Scarecrow Press, 1982. p. 110.

[31] Grove, Pearce S., and Clement, Evelyn G., eds. Bibliographic Control of Nonprint Media. Chicago, American Library Association, 1972. p. 163-165.

[32] AVLINE. National Library of Medicine, 8600 Rockville Pike, Bethesda, Maryland.

[33] Reference List of Audiovisual Materials Produced by the United States Government. National Audiovisual Center, National Archives and Records Service. U.S. General Services Administration, 1978. 388 p. Supplement, 1980. 90 p.

[34]Londos, Eutychia G. Productions and Publications in Health Sciences Audiovisuals of the United States Government: A History 1893-1982. Springfield, Ill. Illinois Libraries. [Spring Special Issue], [1982]. [40] p.

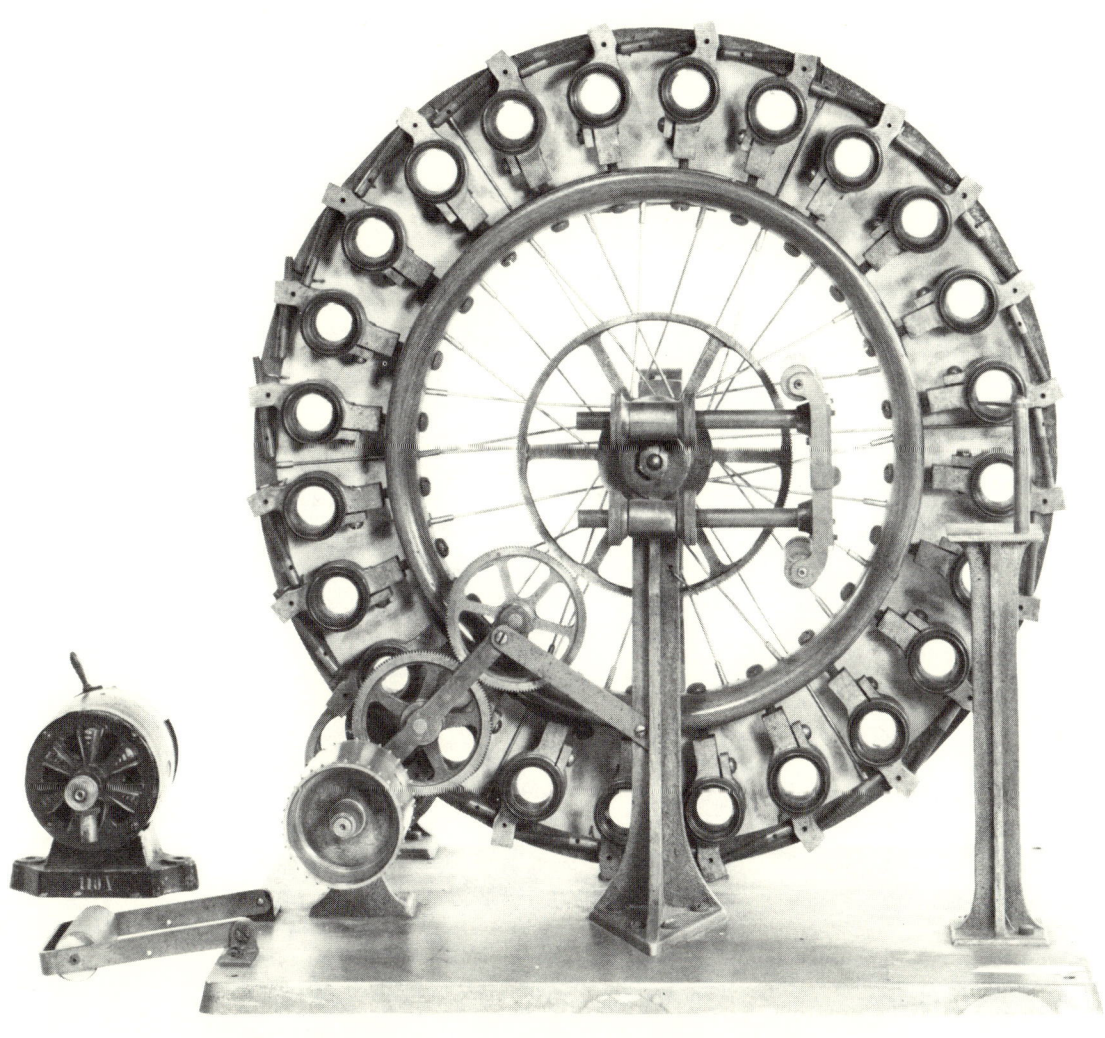

PLATE I. JENKIN'S MOTION PICTURE CAMERA: 1894
ROTARY LENS APPARATUS

Courtesy of The History of Photographic Collection, Smithsonian Institution (reproduced).

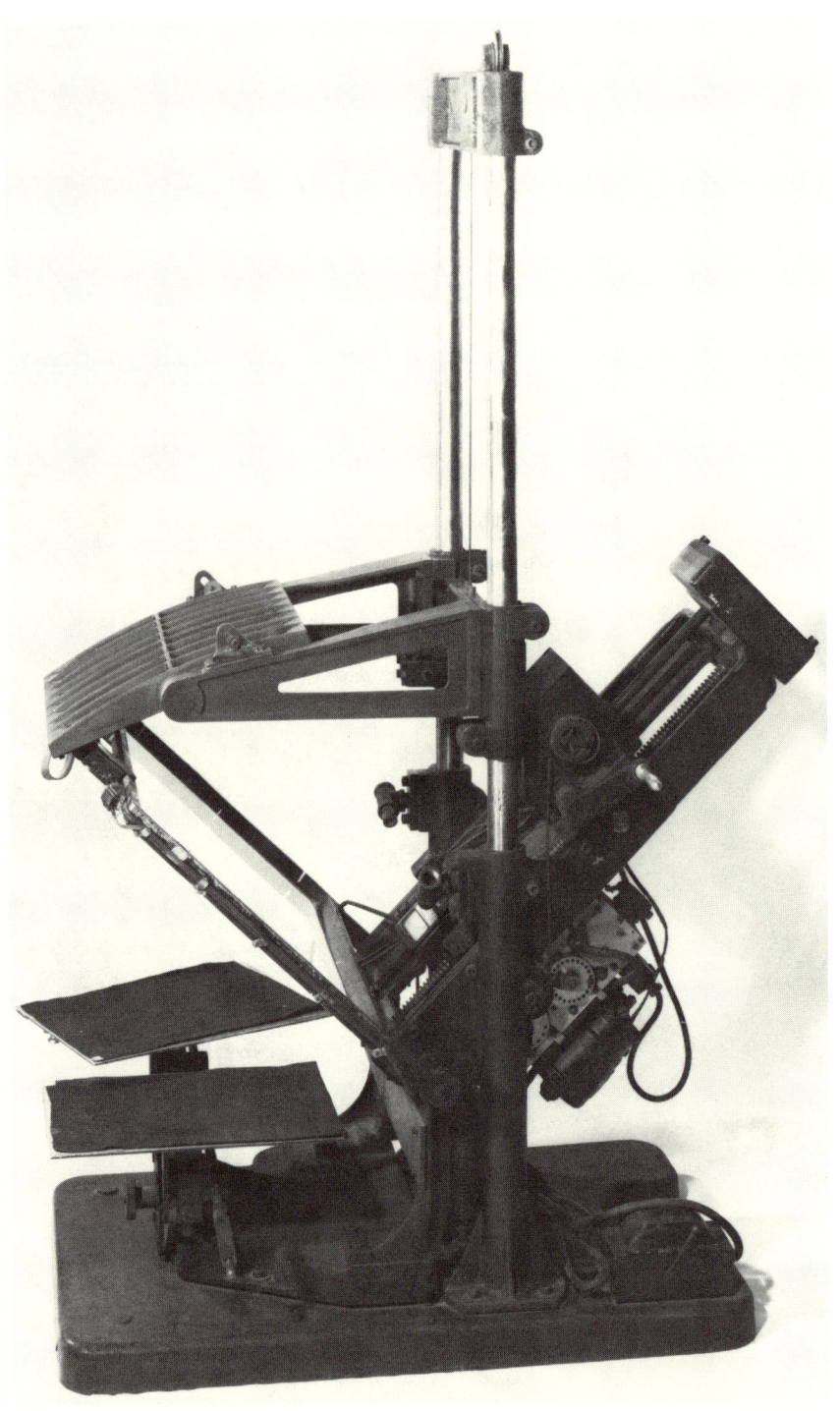

PLATE II. DREAGER MICROFILM CAMERA: 1933-1935

Designed by Lt. R.H. Draeger, USN, 1935-37; automatic focusing, platens automatically adjust to book thickness as pages are turned, semi-automatic operations; 200' film magazine. Gift of Science Service, Inc.

Courtesy of the History of Photographic Collection, Smithsonian Institution.
Source: Armed Forces Medical Library (reproduced).

Publications

ADULT GROUP LEADER GUIDE for USE WITH DIAL A-L-C-O-H-O-L and JACKSON JUNIOR HIGH: TWO FILM SERIES on ALCOHOL EDUCATION

National Institute on Alcohol Abuse and Alcoholism, Office of Education. U.S. Department of Health, Education, and Welfare. 1977. 48 p.

(This guide was prepared by the Abt Associates, Inc. for the National Institute of Alcohol Abuse and Alcoholism. Peter Finn, editor et al.)

MEDIA	16mm films, videocassettes.
SUMMARY	This *Guide* is designed to enable users to use the four DIAL A-L-C-O-H-O-L and four *Jackson Junior High* films with maximum effect. Although the films were originally designed by junior and senior high school students, every film can be used as an enriching and stimulating experience for adult audience depending on the groups. Includes eight film series divided into two groups: Jackson Junior High series entitled 1) Route One, 2) The Party's Over, 3) Barbara Murray, 4) Like Father, Like Son? DIAL A-L-C-O-H-O-L: 1) Hotline, 2) In the Beginning, 3) Al's Garage, 4) The Legend of Paulie Green. Topics or issues covered in these series are: abstinence, alcohol's passage through the body, alcoholism/problem drinking, attitude formation, behavioral and physical effects, children with an alcoholic parent, drinking and driving, drinking customs/history, drunkenness, family drinking problems, helping problem drinkers/alcoholics/legal drinking age, misconceptions about alcohol, parents' role vis-a-vis children drinking, peer pressure, pleasures of drinking, problem drinking/alcoholism, religious issues, reasons social drinkers drink, responsibility for other people with drinking problems, risk taking, teaching methods, teenage drinking, women and alcohol. "For the widest distribution of the television and film alcohol education program, the U.S. Office of Education obtained all clearances on the films and curriculum materials and encourages their reproduction for unlimited future use." (Ordering information section) For information contact the Alcohol TV Project Officer, Room 3116, ROB-3, U.S. Office of Education, Washington, D.C. 20202, (202) 245-9228.
ENTRIES	Film number, title, synopsis, goals, additional annotation on specific subject areas covered by the program. Format, running time, film ordering number, availability, and price are given in the *Ordering Information* section.
SPECIAL FEATURES	Includes information on the purposes of the programs, bibliography of additional print materials, a list of organizations dealing with alcohol, and pictures related to the programs.

ORDERING INFORMATION Available from the Superintendent of Documents, U.S. Government Printing Office Stock No. 017-080-01773-3.

PRICE $2.30. School personnel may write for free loan brochure to NCALI, Department OE, Box 2345, Rockville, Maryland 20852.

AoA CATALOG of FILMS on AGING

Administration on Aging, Social Rehabilitation Service. U.S. Department of Health, Education, and Welfare. 1973. 59 p. Plus announcements.

MEDIA	8mm, 16mm, 35mm, filmstrips, videocassettes, slides, TV spots.
SUMMARY	Includes approximately 110 audiovisual materials dealing with many subjects in the field of aging. These audiovisuals are produced by U.S. Government agencies, universities, associations, independent and commercial producers. Categories include: health care (in-home services, community facilities, institutional medical care), health—preventive services (nutrition, safety), health—rehabilitation, income, living arrangements, retirement (preparation, roles and activities). The General Films section includes materials concerned with aging "per se—its benefits and problems, contributions and needs. They depict the attitudes of society toward its older members—some show the negative outlook... while others take a positive slant, illustrating various ways of meeting needs, adjusting to new life and enjoying a new type of freedom in retirement" (Introduction). Some of the materials date back to 1950.
ENTRIES	Title, annotation, format, color or b/w, sound or silent, running time or number of frames, year of release (if available), producer, distributor, free loan information, rental and purchase, additional information on producer and distributor.
SPECIAL FEATURES	Includes title index.
ORDERING INFORMATION	Available from the Superintendent of Documents, U.S. Government Printing Office. Stock Number 1762-00071.
PRICE	$3.95. Single copy free from the Administration on Aging.

ARMY FILMS for NON-PROFIT USE

U.S. Army. Fifth Headquarters (Fort Sam Houston, Tx.). 1972. 92 p. Plus special announcements.

MEDIA	16mm films.
SUMMARY	Includes approximately 1,000 audiovisual entries for public use. Many films are classified as "historical" while others "restricted" but most are available to civic, religious, fraternal and educational groups, schools, colleges and universities, and other agencies interested in non-profit showing of these films. Broad subject areas covered are biological/chemical/radiological elements as part of combat atmosphere, dentistry, dermatology, emergency evacuation procedures, energy, explosives and safety, hematology, medical effects of nuclear radiation fallout, medical examination, natural disaster, neurology, nursing, obstetrics, occupational health, occupational therapy, personal hygiene, prevention of injuries, speech and hearing problems, surgery, X-rays.
ENTRIES	Prefix and number of film, title, color or b/w, running time, annotation, audience level(s), year of release (when available), distribution information.
SPECIAL FEATURES	Includes a list of area services, information on availability of films, and order form.
ORDERING INFORMATION	Available from the Headquarters Fifth United States Army, Fort Sam Houston, Texas. Fifth U.S. Army Pamphlet 108-1.
PRICE	Free.

AUDIO-VISUAL MATERIALS CATALOG—ARTHRITIS INFORMATION CLEARINGHOUSE

National Institute of Arthritis, Metabolism, and Digestive Diseases, National Institutes of Health, Public Health Service. U.S. Department of Health and Human Services. April 1981. 95 p.

MEDIA	16mm films, filmstrips with audiotapes, videocassettes, slide sets with audiotapes, audiotapes, film cartridges, audiotapes with microfiche, magnetic tapes, microfiche.
SUMMARY	Includes both print and nonprint materials produced by U.S. Government agencies, independent producers, medical schools, and foundations concerning all aspects in the field of arthritis. The 250 audiovisual entries are classified under 180 subject headings. Broad subject categories are: diagnosis and treatment, drug therapy and side effects, employment and legal aspects, etiology, nutrition/diet, prevention, rehabilitation, research, study cases, voluntary health agencies. Some audiovisuals are in Spanish.
ENTRIES	Accession number, author (when available), title, producer, format, year of release, coursebook, color or b/w, sound or silent, running time, annotation, distributor's address, order number, sale price, primary audience, number of references.
SPECIAL FEATURES	Includes the following indexes: title, subject, format, primary audience, source. Appendix of related print materials is also included.
ORDERING INFORMATION	Available from the Arthritis Information Clearinghouse. NIH Publication No. 80-2380.
PRICE	Free.

AUDIOVISUAL AIDS DIRECTORY of the REHABILITATION RESEARCH and TRAINING CENTERS: AUDIOTAPE, FILM, SLIDES, VIDEOTAPE. Second Edition.

Rehabilitation Services Administration, Office of Human Development. U.S. Department of Health, Education and Welfare. 1975. 229 p.

(This publication was prepared by Irvin C. Mohler and Jared Sonies, Science Communication Division, Department of Medical and Public Affairs, The George Washington University Medical Center, Washington, D.C., in cooperation with the George Washington University Rehabilitation Research and Training Center (RT-9). Work supported by Grant SRS-16-P-56803/3-11. GS-SCD 75-09P.)

MEDIA	16mm films, videocassettes, slide sets, audiotapes, transparencies.
SUMMARY	This directory represents an up-to-date compilation of 566 audiovisual materials developed by the R&T Centers and others for use in training and teaching programs and are available on a loan, rental, purchase or duplication basis. These audiovisuals which are classified under 250 subject headings represent the following broad subject areas: alcohol and alcoholism, amputation, anatomy, arthritis, behaviour modification/hyperactivity, body mechanics, cancer care, cardiovascular, cerebral palsy, community activities, counseling, death and dying, dentistry, diet, Down's syndrome, drug abuse, drug therapy, employment/vocational rehabilitation, epilepsy, equipment/homemaking and self-help devices, ethnic groups, federal and state programs, genetics, gerontology, hypoxia, mental retardation, neurology, nursing, nutrition, pain/diagnosis and treatment, physical fitness, physical medicine, physiology, psychiatry and psychology, public health, pulmonary disorders, rehabilitation, research, sex education, social work, surgery, urinary tract, vocational training.
ENTRIES	AV number (indicating format), title, annotation, format, producer/sponsor, target audience, recommended follow-up, running time, color or b/w, sound or silent, equipment specification, accompanying print materials, availability, rental, loan, purchase, or duplication cost, source.
SPECIAL FEATURES	The directory is divided into chapters, with each chapter representing one R&T Center. Audiovisuals for each Center are grouped into four categories: audiotape or disc; film, slide; overhead transparency or filmstrip; and videotape. It includes the addresses of the research and training centers, a title index, index of lecturers, a subject index, and information to the users.

ORDERING INFORMATION	Available from the Rehabilitation Services Administration.
PRICE	Free.

AUDIOVISUAL AIDS for HIGH BLOOD PRESSURE EDUCATION

National High Blood Pressure Education Program, National Heart, Lung, and Blood Institute, National Institutes of Health, Public Health Service. U.S. Department of Health, Education, and Welfare. October 1979. 95 p. Plus supplements and announcements.

MEDIA	16mm films, filmstrips, videocassettes, slide sets, audiocassettes.
SUMMARY	This mediagraphy contains 150 audiovisual entries designed to further efforts of high blood pressure control by providing medical personnel with the tools they need to continue their own education and instruct their patients and the general public. These entries are produced no earlier than 1974, but a few entries produced since 1970 are included because either they are in Spanish or the production date is not available. The catalog is divided into three main sections: Public Education, Patient Education, and Professional Education. These are further subdivided into following subject area categories and treatment methods: children and adolescents, compliance, diet, drug treatment, epidemiology, evaluation and diagnosis, hypertensive emergencies, management of high blood pressure, measurement of blood pressure, mechanisms, obstetrics/gynecology, organ damage, other (includes hypertension series for nurses), secondary hypertension. These entries are produced by both the U.S. Government agencies and independent producers.
ENTRIES	Title, consultant, producer, year of release, annotation, format, recommended audience, ordering information.
SPECIAL FEATURES	Includes title and subject indexes, lists of distributors and producers, users' assessment form.
ORDERING INFORMATION	Available from the High Blood Pressure Information Center, 120/80 National Institutes of Health. NIH Publication No. 80-1663, October 1979. U.S. Government Printing Office: 1980 0-634-975.
PRICE	$4.45. Single copy free from the High Blood Pressure Information Center.

AUDIOVISUAL CATALOG — NIDA RESOURCE CENTER

National Institute on Drug Abuse Resource Center. (Department of Health and Human Services, Public Health Service, Alcohol Drug Abuse, and Mental Health Administration). 1980. [32] p.

MEDIA	8mm and/or 16mm films, filmstrips, videocassettes, audiotapes, kits, recordings, games.
SUMMARY	This catalog contains approximately 360 audiovisual materials on the following subjects: community programs, counseling, crisis series, criminal justice, DIAL A-L-C-O-H-O-L series, drugs and drug addiction, government treatment programs, mental health, prevention, smoking, teacher training, and treatment. These audiovisuals are available for loan to individuals and groups.
ENTRIES	Title, accession number, format.
SPECIAL FEATURES	Includes the DIAL A-L-C-O-H-O-L series. Information on other services by the NIDA Resource Center is also included.
ORDERING INFORMATION	Available from the U.S. Government Printing Office: [1980] 0-274-043.
PRICE	Free.

AUDIOVISUAL CATALOG of the NATIONAL HIGHWAY TRAFFIC SAFETY ADMINISTRATION — December 1970-December 1973. Plus announcements.

National Highway Traffic Safety Administration. U.S. Department of Transportation. 1974. 846 p. Plus announcements.

(Distribution through the National Highway Traffic Safety Administration is indefinitely discontinued. Audiovisuals are temporarily available from the National Audiovisual Center and/or The National Safety Council.)

MEDIA	16mm films, slide sets, still photographs.
SUMMARY	The 4,000 audiovisual entries listed in this catalog which were produced by the National Highway Traffic Safety Administration (NHTFA) represent all aspects of the auto industry and safety on a national and international level. Broad health sciences categories included are: alcohol related accidents, AMA studies on accidents and their causes, aviation medicine, biological and physiological factors in accidents, court depositions of cases, death and injury statistics, environmental problems related to moving vehicles, impact of licit and illicit drugs on driving, industrial safety and health, law enforcement and court cases, medical investigations on accidents, safety design, research in auto industry. The catalog is divided into two sections: catalog index where entries are arranged by sequential number reflecting their arrangement on the shelf in the Technical Services Division, and KWIC (or keyword) index where each significant word in the title entry is displayed in an alphabetical order in the center column of the page—under the heading "Keyword." Audiovisuals are available to the public on a free loan basis.
ENTRIES	Catalog index section: entries are arranged by their sequential number reflecting the arrangement of the audiovisuals on the shelf in the Technical Services Division, followed by the number given by the contractor or other agencies involved in the contract reports, contractor or organization responsible for the production, contract number and other internal reporting symbols, title, year of production, number of copies available, restrictions (if any), running time, format, color or b/w, sound or silent. KWIC index section: entries are arranged by keyword reflecting their alphabetical order. This section also functions as subject index.
SPECIAL FEATURES	Includes detailed explanation for catalog arrangement, and a sample of Technical Report Documentation. A keyword section provides a subject index.

ORDERING   Available from the National Technical Information Service (NTIS) DOT
INFORMATION   HS-801 212.

PRICE $15.00.

AUDIOVISUAL GUIDE to the CATALOG of the FOOD and NUTRITION INFORMATION and EDUCATIONAL MATERIALS CENTER

Food and Nutrition Information and Educational Materials Center, National Agricultural Library. U.S. Department of Agriculture. 2nd edition. 1977. 132 p. Plus announcement.

MEDIA	16mm films, filmstrips, videocassettes, slide sets, audiotapes, transparencies, film loops, charts, games, recordings, kits, food models, metric converters, nutrimeters, study prints.
SUMMARY	This catalog includes 800 audiovisual materials classified under an equal number of subject headings, covering all phases of food and nutrition. Materials produced by both U.S. Government agencies and independent producers from around the world, including the United Nations Food and Agriculture Organization (UNFAO), are all available from the Center. Broad subject categories are: agriculture, career guidance, child feeding, community health, dental health, diet, food preparation, gardening, industry, nutrition, obesity, pesticides, physiology, pregnancy and infant feeding, quackery and technology, sanitation, teaching methods, tobacco, vitamins, world food problems. Most of the audiovisuals are current but some date back to 1950.
ENTRIES	Accession number, title, format, edition, producer(s), running time or number of frames, color or b/w, year of release, subject(s), accompanying print material(s), annotation, series.
SPECIAL FEATURES	This catalog includes the following additional information: Center's other services available to the public, a list of catalogs and supplements published by the Center, computer retrieval services, audiovisual glossary, information on audiovisual equipment, subject, author and corporate author indexes, and information on availability of the Center's magnetic tapes.
ORDERING INFORMATION	Available from the Superintendent of Documents, U.S. Government Printing Office: 1977 720-069/6853. The catalog is also available on magnetic tape. Tapes are standard half-inch, 9 track, 800 or 1600 bpi, in EBCDIC, with standard IBM headers and trailers. Records are variable length from 1973 to 3878 characters, blocked 2.
PRICE	Tape: [$45.00 per reel]. Print: $9.95.

AUDIOVISUAL MATERIALS in DENTAL AUXILIARY EDUCATION

Learning Resources Branch, Bureau of Health Manpower, Health Resources Administration, Public Health Service. U.S. Department of Health, Education, and Welfare. 1975. 192 p.

MEDIA
: 8mm and/or 16mm films, filmstrips, videocassettes, Kinescope (video), slide sets, audiotapes, transparencies, recordings.

SUMMARY
: Lists and describes 922 available audiovisual materials in dental auxiliary education. Three sections are included in the catalog: Subject-Title Index with audiovisual materials indexed and cross-indexed under 48 teaching areas; Descriptions of Audiovisual Materials with complete description arranged alphabetically by first significant word of the title; and Distributor List with names and complete addresses of organizations and their collections included in the compilation. Some titles appeared in earlier publication, *Audiovisual Materials in Dental Education, 1973*. The materials included have been evaluated for currency and effectiveness. Includes materials produced by U.S. Government agencies, commercial distributors and producers, and professional associations. Materials that have been evaluated favorably are available through the information exchange, AVLINE (Audiovisuals On-Line), U.S. National Library of Medicine (NLM). Subjects included are: anatomy (oral), anesthesiology, articulation, asepsis/sterilization, cancer (oral), caries (dental), chairside assisting, community dentistry, crown and bridge, dental assisting, dental laboratory technology, dental materials, embryology, endodontics, ethics/jurisprudence, examination/diagnosis/treatment, expanded functions, fluoridation, histology, hospital dentistry, impression taking, in-service education, instrumentation, morphology, nutrition, occlusion, operative/restorative, orthodontics, pathology (oral), patient education, patient management, pedodontics, periodontics, plaque control/removal, practice administration/management, preventive dentistry, prosthodontics, radiology/photography, recruitment, rubber dam application, scaling/planning/curettage, special patient care, and other subject areas such as blood coagulation, dental drug interactions, operation and maintenance of dental units, prescription writing in dentistry, story of Dr. Lister (The)—16mm film, technique in venipuncture, and Weber Unit chair instruction. Film entries have been produced beginning in 1950 to the present.

ENTRIES
: Title, producer/author (when available), year of release, running time or number of frames, format, silent or sound, color or b/w, accompanying print material(s), distributor, annotation.

SPECIAL FEATURES	Includes Subject-Title Index, Distributors List, and information on restrictions on materials considered for inclusion in the catalog and on the use of these materials.
ORDERING INFORMATION	Superintendent of Documents, U.S. Government Printing Office: 1976-641-307/4513 Region No. 4, HRA Publication No. 76-86.
PRICE	$6.50.

BIMONTHLY LIST of PUBLICATIONS and AUDIOVISUALS

Office of Communications. U.S. Department of Agriculture. 1961- . (Title varies slightly)

(This publication is located in all Depository Libraries. For individual issues, write to the Office of Communications, U.S. Department of Agriculture. Individual issues are free to the public.)

MEDIA	16mm films, filmstrips, slide sets.
SUMMARY	This publication includes both print and nonprint materials on a free loan basis or on a low cost rental to the public. It is designed to assist individuals to locate materials concerning agriculture. All materials included are published/produced by the U.S. Department of Agriculture. Audiovisuals are listed in the special section "Motion Pictures" covering broad subjects. Specific subject areas included are: activities of the Horticultural Society, environment, farming, fire safety, food and nutrition, forest diseases, fruit and gardening, herpetology, history of the development of American agriculture, national emergency during epidemics of sleeping sickness, plant diseases, poultry, recreation, soil and water conservation, vegetation, war against pests, weather, wildlife and game.
ENTRIES	Title, year of release, running time or number of frames, format, sound or silent, color or b/w, annotation.
SPECIAL FEATURES	Includes publications related to audiovisuals and agriculture. Order form is also included.
ORDERING INFORMATION	See above.
PRICE	Individual issues free (see above).

CANCER FILM GUIDE 1963

Cancer Control Branch, Division of Chronic Diseases, Public Health Service. U.S. Department of Health, Education, and Welfare. 1963. 183 p.

MEDIA	16mm films.
SUMMARY	Includes 1,510 motion pictures relating to cancer to assist medical schools, hospitals, and other users in their quest for teaching materials. These materials are arranged in 103 categories. Broad subject categories are: abdomen and pelvis, adrenal gland, biliary tract and pancreas, bladder and uterus, blood, bones, brain and spinal cord, breast cancer (general), chemotherapy, child, colon and rectum, diagnosis (general), esophagus, eye and eyelids, head and neck, heart, kidney, larynx, lung and bronchi, lymph and genitalia, mouth, tongue and lips, parotid gland, radiology, research, skin, small intestine, spleen, stomach, thorax and mediastinum, thyroid gland, uterus and cervix uteri, vulva and vagina.
ENTRIES	Title, sponsor or producer, year of release, agency, country of origin, sound or silent, color or b/w, running time, format, annotation, credits, distributor.
SPECIAL FEATURES	Includes distributor list, list of categories, and subject listing.
ORDERING INFORMATION	Available from the National Technical Information Service (NTIS) PHS Publication No. 848.
PRICE	$3.50.

CAREER EDUCATION: SELECTED U.S. GOVERNMENT AUDIOVISUALS

National Audiovisual Center, National Archives and Records Service. U.S. General Services Administration. October 1977. 59 p.

MEDIA	16mm films, filmstrips, videocassettes, slide sets, audiotapes, multimedia kits, recordings.
SUMMARY	This directory includes approximately 400 audiovisual entries produced by U.S. Government agencies since 1965 dealing with careers in the following fields: aviation, emergency technicians, food, health services, marines, medical technicians, meteorology in the navy, nursing, nuclear sciences, oceanic sciences, personal hygiene, veterinary sciences, and youth programs.
ENTRIES	Title, format, running time or number of frames, year of release, rental or purchase information, annotation, TV clearance, note on use of audiovisuals and producer(s).
SPECIAL FEATURES	Gives information on other catalogs published by the National Audiovisual Center, ordering information, and information on public services by the Center.
ORDERING INFORMATION	Available from the National Audiovisual Center.
PRICE	Free.

CASSETTE BOOKS

Division for the Blind and Physically Handicapped. U.S. Library of Congress. 1975-. Bimonthly.

MEDIA	Cassettes.
SUMMARY	A network of cooperating libraries throughout the country lends books and magazines from the Library of Congress Program collection free of charge. Readers may also receive cassette machines and phonographs on indefinite loan. This catalog lists all cassette books produced by the Division for the Blind and Physically Handicapped. The magazine is divided into sections to include areas such as adult nonfiction, adult fiction, young adult, and all topics on liberal arts and sciences. Medicine and health areas are also included. (See also *Catalog of Educational Films for the Deaf 1980-81.*)
ENTRIES	Title, author, narrator(s), identification number, annotation, year of publication.
SPECIAL FEATURES	Includes information on The Division for the Blind and Physcially Handicapped's activities, information on how to use the system, eligibility, ordering information, surveys, and related print materials. Order form is also included.
ORDERING INFORMATION	Available from the cooperating public library in the area. For additional information write to: Publication Services, Division for the Blind and Physically Handicapped, Library of Congress, Washington, D.C. 20542.
PRICE	Distributed free of charge to participants in the Library of Congress Cassette Books for the Handicapped.

CATALOG of AUDIO-VISUAL AIDS in HYPERTENSION

High Blood Pressure Information Center, National Institutes of Health, Public Health Services. U.S. Department of Health, Education, and Welfare. 1975. 110 p.

MEDIA	16mm films, videocassettes, slide sets, audiocassettes.
SUMMARY	Includes approximately 75 annotated entries produced by government agencies, independent producers, professional associations, and pharmaceutical companies dealing with problems in hypertension. Its comprehensive coverage includes community programs, diagnosis and treatment, and epidemiology. Workshops for the laymen and professionals are also included. The catalog is divided into six sections: General public: patient education. Professional: educating the patient. Professional: essential hypertension, detection, diagnosis, and treatment. Professional: secondary hypertension. All materials are available from various distributors given in each entry.
ENTRIES	Title, producer, author (when applicable), annotation, running time or number of frames, format, color or b/w, sound or silent, recommended use, order number, availability source, producer's address, rental and purchase information, previewer, additional materials.
SPECIAL FEATURES	Includes name and address of producer and distributor for each individual entry.
ORDERING INFORMATION	Available from the National Heart, Lung, and Blood Institute No. 1975 0-574-596.
PRICE	Free.

CATALOG of EDUCATIONAL CAPTIONED FILMS for the DEAF 1980-81

U.S. Department of Education. Prepared by the Special Materials Project of the Association for Education on the Deaf. 1980. 175 p.

(Funds for publication of this catalog were provided by Captioned Films and Telecommunications Branch, Office of Special Education and Rehabilitation Services.)

MEDIA	16mm films (captioned).
SUMMARY	Contains annotated entries for 2,000 captioned films for use in instructional and entertainment programs for the deaf. These films were produced by either U.S. Government agencies or by independent producers in the United States and abroad. All entries are selected by the Captioned Films and Telecommunications Branch of the Office of Special Education, and redistributed free of charge to schools and classes for the deaf through 60 distribution centers. This well-organized and detailed catalog has two principle parts: subject index, and alphabetical list of captioned films descriptions which lists films by subject headings and by titles. Among the subjects included in the broad categories are: animals/zoology, career education, consumer education, fine arts and crafts, guidance, health and safety, hygiene, language arts, mathematics, physical education, science, social studies. Materials are available to all schools and associations registered with the distributing centers. "A free national library service providing braille and recorded materials for blind and physically handicapped persons is administered by the Library of Congress Division for the Blind and Physically Handicapped. With copyright permission granted by authors and publishers, the Library of Congress selects and produces full-length books and magazines in braille and on recorded disc and cassette. These books and magazines are then distributed to a cooperating network of 56 regional and nearly 100 subregional (local) libraries that circulate them to eligible borrowers. Reading materials are sent to readers and returned to libraries by postage-free mail. Established by an act of Congress in 1931 to serve blind adults, this program was expanded in 1952 to include children, and again in 1966 by Public Law 89-522 to include individuals with other physical impairments that prevent the reading of standard print." (Division for the Blind and Physically Handicapped, Library of Congress *Fact Sheet, Books for the Blind and Physically Handicapped.* April 1977.)
ENTRIES	Title, captioned film number, running time, color or b/w, SYNCAP (indicating that the sound track of the film is synchronized with the captions), annotation, series titles, subject heading(s), interest levels, producer/distributor, production date or year of release, lesson guide (referring to the edition of the lesson guide when additional information can be obtained), and page number in lesson guide.

SPECIAL FEATURES	Includes brief history and use of captioned films, 1958 Public Law Act, instruction to borrowers, care of films, inservice training packet outline, utilization of captioned film lesson guides, glossary of common terms, key to captioned film descriptions, list of distributors other than governmental, special instructions to borrowers, and accession listing of films. Lists of withdrawn films and additional educational titles are also included. There is also an invitation with special instructions to those who wish to participate in the production of captioned films.
ORDERING INFORMATION	Available from the Superintendent of Documents, U.S. Government Printing Office: 1980 334.971.7017. For participation in distribution write for an account number to: Special Materials Project, Captioned Films for the Deaf Distribution Center, 814 Thayler Avenue, Silver Springs, Maryland 20910.
PRICE	Single copy free from the Special Materials Project.
SEE ALSO:	BRAILLE BOOK REVIEW, CASSETTE BOOKS, CATALOG OF TRAINING FILMS AND OTHER MEDIA FOR SPECIAL EDUCATION, HEALTH: A SELECTED LIST OF BOOKS THAT HAVE APPEARED IN TALKING BOOKS TOPICS AND BRAILLE BOOK REVIEW, and TALKING BOOK TOPICS included in this publication.

CATALOG of FAMILY PLANNING MATERIALS

Bureau of Community Health, Health Services Administration, Public Health Service. U.S. Department of Health, Education, and Welfare. 1979. 144 p.

MEDIA	8mm, 16mm, 32mm films, filmstrips, videocassettes, slide sets, audio-cassettes, multimedia kits.
SUMMARY	Includes approximately 650 audiovisuals produced by both government agencies and independent producers, covering a wide variety of topics on family planning. These materials are arranged under the following sections: Family Planning, Related Topics, Materials for the Professional, Miscellaneous Materials. Under those sections the materials are arranged under their subjects. Specific subjects covered are: adolescents, adoption, birth defects and genetics, contraceptive methods, health and health services, handicapped, human sexuality, infertility, knowledge/attitudes/practice, reproduction and reproductive systems, sex education, sterilization, and venereal diseases. Breast cancer, cancer in men, pharmaceuticals (drug therapy), hotlines, and youth crisis lines are also included. In the miscellaneous section, bumper stickers, posters, and models are included. Most of the entries are produced within the last ten years. The majority of the audiovisuals are available in Spanish.
ENTRIES	Title, language, distributor, year of release, format, color or b/w, running time or number of frames, purchase and rental price (when applicable), annotation, series, and accompanying print material(s).
ORDERING INFORMATION	Available from the Superintendent of Documents, U.S. Government Printing Office: 1979–623-013/6662. DHEW Publication No. (HSA) 79-5606, 1979.
PRICE	$3.25.

CATALOG of FILMS AVAILABLE from AGENCIES: The U.S. DEPARTMENT of COMMERCE SERVING the NATION

U.S. Department of Commerce. [1979] 19 p.

MEDIA	16mm films, slide sets.
SUMMARY	Includes 68 audiovisual materials produced by the following U.S. Government agencies: The Bureau of the Census, Maritime Administration, National Bureau of Standards, National Oceanic and Atmospheric Administration, and the Office of Energy Programs. Subjects covered by the audiovisuals are: animal life, biology, chemistry, energy, fire safety, law enforcement equipment standards, lead and paint poisoning, marine biology, natural disaster programs, noise control, physical education, population statistics, port preparedness in case of natural disaster or enemy attacks, and recreation. Most of the materials are current, but some of them date back to 1950. All entries are available for public use from the Association-Sterling Films, the U.S. Department of Commerce District Offices, or from the National Audiovisual Center (NAC).
ENTRIES	Title, running time, annotation, availability, intended audience, ordering information, rental or purchase price (where applicable).
SPECIAL FEATURES	Provides lists of the Association-Sterling Films Libraries and the U.S. Department of Commerce Offices. Gives information on free loan films directly from the U.S. Department of Commerce.
ORDERING INFORMATION	Available from the U.S. Department of Commerce, Office of Communications.
PRICE	Free.

CATALOG of the FDA PUBLICATIONS and AUDIOVISUAL MATERIALS for CONSUMERS

Food and Drug Administration, Public Health Service. U.S. Department of Health, Education, and Welfare. 1977. 29 p.

MEDIA	16mm films, slide sets, table-top exhibits, quizmatic exhibits.
SUMMARY	Includes both publications and audiovisuals. Publications are available free to the public through the nearest FDA Consumer Affairs Officer or directly from Consumer Inquiries, Food and Drug Administration. Twenty audiovisuals are primarily used by the FDA Consumer Affairs Officers in presentations to consumer groups or at conventions, fairs, and smaller events. The catalog is divided into six subject areas: cosmetics, drugs, electronic products that emit radiation, food, medical devices, pharmacology, and prescription and nonprescription drugs. Some programs are in Spanish. For use of audiovisuals the user is instructed to contact the nearest FDA Consumer Affairs Officer for arranging a showing or use of the materials.
ENTRIES	Arranged by title under their format (Films, Slides): title, annotation, format, color or b/w, running time or number of frames. Exhibits: complete display.
SPECIAL FEATURES	A list of the names of the Food and Drug Administration Consumer Affairs Officers around the country by state is included. Print materials related to the audiovisuals are also included in this publication.
ORDERING INFORMATION	Available from the Office of Public Affairs, Food and Drug Administration. DHEW Publication No. (FDA) 77-1030, U.S. Government Printing Office: 1977 0-242-735.
PRICE	Free. Copies of the publication can be obtained either through the nearest FDA Affairs Officer or by writing to Consumer Inquiries, Food and Drug Administration.

CATALOG of the UNITED STATES COAST GUARD FILMS

U.S. Coast Guard. U.S. Department of Transportation. [1975]. 15 p.

MEDIA	16mm films.
SUMMARY	Lists 26 films which present the operations and programs of the U.S. Coast Guard to promote maritime safety, protection, and the saving of lives and property at sea or in the navigable waters of the United States. Entries are divided into two categories: general interest films, and boating safety films. Specific subject areas covered by the films are: AMVER (Automated Mutual-assistance Vessel Rescue system) and its medical capability in disaster cases, films on the role of the Coast Guard personnel in the early days on Mississippi, Missouri, and Ohio rivers, environmental problems, firefighting, food operations, port security, recreation, search and rescue operations, and training of personnel. The film entries have been produced beginning in 1944 to the present.
ENTRIES	Title, color or b/w, running time, year of release, TV clearance, producer, film number.
SPECIAL FEATURES	Provides information on special services of the U.S. Coast Guard, list of U.S. Coast Guard Libraries for public use, and pictures. Indexes on general interest films, and boating safety films are also included.
ORDERING INFORMATION	Available from the U.S. Department of Transportation, U.S. Coast Guard.
PRICE	Free.

CATALOG of TRAINING FILMS and OTHER MEDIA for SPECIAL EDUCATION

Division of Media Services, Bureau of Education for the Handicapped, Office of Education. U.S. Department of Health, Education, and Welfare. January, 1977. 30 p.

(This publication was prepared by the Special Office for Materials Distribution.)

SUMMARY	This catalog includes approximately 300 instructional materials designed to be used by professionals in special education for pre- and inservice training. Organizations, institutions or agencies training individuals to work with the handicapped; businesses and agencies employing the handicapped or interested in hiring the handicapped; and schools, classes, rehabilitation centers, and other educational groups working with the handicapped are eligible users. Subjects included are: adjustment, art/training methods, audiology, behavior disorders and modification, blindness, cerebral palsy, classroom management, communication/deaf, creativity, deaf-blind, diagnosis, early childhood, education/Europe, emotional disturbance, evaluation techniques, fingerspelling, geography, handicapped children, hearing impairment, instruction/inner city/design, integration, language, mental retardation, Montessori, multiple handicaps, parent education, physical education, Piaget, reading, sciences, special education, speech, visual impairment. (See also *Catalog of Educational Films for the Deaf 1980-81*)
SPECIAL FEATURES	Includes a detailed information section for the users, alphabetical list of subject headings and see references, and subject heading index.
ORDERING INFORMATION	Available from the Division of Media Services, Bureau for the Handicapped, U.S. Office of Education.
PRICE	Free.

CHILD ABUSE and NEGLECT AUDIOVISUAL MATERIALS

National Center on Child Abuse and Neglect, Children's Bureau, Administration for Children, Youth and Family, Office of Human Development Services. U.S. Department of Health and Human Services. May 1980. 92 p.

(This publication was developed by Herner and Company under Contract Number HEW-105-78-1101 for National Center on Child Abuse and Neglect, Children's Bureau.)

MEDIA	16mm films, videocassettes, slide sets, multimedia kits.
SUMMARY	The National Center on Child Abuse and Neglect gathers and disseminates information concerning all aspects of child abuse and neglect. This catalog contains audiovisuals identified through a variety of sources, which were donated to the Center by child abuse and neglect programs throughout the country. Includes 345 current entries reviewed and recommended which are classified under the following broad subjects: abuse, accidents, behavior modification, community health, counseling, drug abuse, education, ethnic groups, evolution (child development), family planning, government programs, history, Indians, jurisprudence, mental retardation, minority groups, nutrition, organization/management of personnel, pediatrics, public health, social sciences, psychiatry and psychology, sex societies, volunteer services. Some audiovisuals are in Spanish.
ENTRIES	Accession number, producer, title, format, year of release/production (when available), distributor, rental and sale price, annotation.
SPECIAL FEATURES	The entries are grouped under formats, gives names and address of distributors, and includes subject and title indexes.
ORDERING INFORMATION	Available from the Superintendent of Documents, U.S. Government Printing Office, DHHS Publication No. (OHDS) 80-30125.
PRICE	$5.00.

CRIMINAL JUSTICE AUDIOVISUAL MATERIALS DIRECTORY

Audiovisual Communications Division, Office of Operations Support, Law Enforcement Assistance Administration. U.S. Department of Justice. 2nd edition. October 1976. 120 p. Plus supplements.

MEDIA	16mm films, videocassettes, audiotapes.
SUMMARY	This directory is designed as a resource guide to those in the criminal justice field seeking materials for education, training, and orientation. The directory is divided into five sections: Courts (140 entries), Police Techniques and Training (400 entries), Prevention (150 entries), Prisons and Rehabilitation/Corrections (42 entries), and Public Education (450 entries). Subjects covered are: accidents and their prevention, addiction (drugs, alcohol, smoking), child molesting, court cases, community programs, drugs and the law, emergency medical patrol calls, first aid/paramedics, intravenous infusion techniques, life and rehabilitation of inmates, medical research on alcohol effects, police role in wife/child abuse, psychiatry, psychology, shock (techniques), social work in prisons, stress (mental health/absenteeism), surgical removal of scars on prisoners' body, violence. Materials listed can be obtained by referring to the production and distribution sources, both government and commercial, which are included in the directory.
ENTRIES	Title, intended audience, annotation, running time, color or b/w, availability, distributor.
SPECIAL FEATURES	Includes distributors list and evaluation form for the users. Brochures, pamphlets, and "community action" materials are also included.
ORDERING INFORMATION	Available from the Superintendent of Documents, U.S. Government Printing Office: Stock No. 027-000-00436-9.
PRICE	$6.95.

DENTAL TRAINING FILMS

Veterans Administration. VA Medical Center, Washington. March 1979. [194] p.

MEDIA	videocassettes.
SUMMARY	Includes approximately 300 entries produced by U.S. Government agencies, dental and medical schools, and the American Dental Association. The twenty-two subjects representing the materials included in the catalog are: anatomy (oral), articulator systems, complete dentures, dental assisting, dental laboratory technology, dental materials, dental office emergencies, diagnosis/oral pathology, endodontics, esthetics, fixed partial dentures, hospital dentistry, maxillo-facial prosthodontics, occlusion, operative dentistry, radiology (oral), patient education, periodontics, pharmacology, preventive dentistry, removable partial dentures, surgery, and miscellaneous entries such as "Sit Down, Doctor—and Live," "The Problem Oriented Medical Record," "Preventive Cross Contamination in Removable Prosthodontics" are also included. The catalog is divided into two sections: section I is a category listing of the films by number and title, indexed according to generalized headings, and section II is a numerical listing of all the currently available films.
ENTRIES	Film number, title, annotation, running time, name of the cooperating author, catalog number of the V.A. issued videocassette which includes that particular program. (See also *Union List of Audiovisuals in the Library Network of the Veterans Administration* and *VA Film Catalog*.)
SPECIAL FEATURES	Includes subject index.
ORDERING INFORMATION	Available from the V.A. Medical Center (Washington, D.C.)
PRICE	Free.

DENTISTRY: A SELECT LIST of U.S. GOVERNMENT PRODUCED AUDIOVISUAL MATERIALS

National Audiovisual Center, National Archives and Records Service, U.S. General Services Administration. 1977. 37 p. Plus announcements.

MEDIA	16mm films, filmstrips, videocassettes, slide sets, audiotapes, recordings.
SUMMARY	These 350 materials for professional training and Continuing Education programs have been produced under the auspices of the U.S. Government over the last ten years. All entries are classified under 16 subject headings. Specific subjects covered are: anatomy and physiology (oral), anesthesiology, cosmetics, dental assistance, training in diagnosis and treatment, emergency care endodontics, nursing and patient care, occlusion, oral hygiene and patient education, oral pathology, oral surgery, periodontics, preventive dentistry, prosthetics, radiology (oral), restorations, and oral cancer.
ENTRIES	Title, running time or number of frames, format, color or b/w, year of release, producer, title number, sale price, annotation, series, accompanying print material(s).
SPECIAL FEATURES	Includes rental and purchase information, policies of the National Audiovisual Center, and title index.
ORDERING INFORMATION	Available from the National Audiovisual Center.
PRICE	Free. (Also available in microfiche from the National Technical Information Service/NTIS) [$3.50]

DIRECTORY of CANCER RESEARCH INFORMATION RESOURCES*

International Cancer Resource Data Bank (ICRDB) Program, National Cancer Institute, National Institutes of Health. U.S. Department of Health, Education, and Welfare. August 1977. 226 p. In various pagings.

MEDIA	16mm films, filmstrips, videocassettes, slide sets, audiotapes, transparencies, recordings, print materials.
SUMMARY	The ICRDB Program was developed in response to a congressional directive in the National Cancer Act of 1971 407(b) (4) which states that the Director of the National Institute of Cancer (NCI) shall: "Collect, analyze, and disseminate all data useful in the prevention, diagnosis, and treatment of cancer, including the establishment of an international cancer research data bank to collect, catalog, store, and disseminate insofar as feasible the results of cancer research undertaken in any country for the use of any person involved in cancer research in any country." (Introduction). This directory provides cancer researchers with a single-volume listing of most of the available cancer information sources around the world. Sources of information range from publications containing research papers through secondary printed and automated sources of abstracts, bibliographies, and synopses of research projects to such diverse services as libraries, audiovisual materials, organizations sponsoring technical meetings and research, cancer registries, government publications, and special information services. It is organized into twelve sections. The twelve sections are further divided into two general groups (publications, and services) as follows: Publications: primary—original research papers and reviews; secondary—bibliographies, abstracts, and indexes to literature; classification schemes—systems of classification of diseases and biomedical information. Services: libraries—primary journals, and other sources of information; special collections—unique oncological material not listed elsewhere; automated service—computer-based information service; audiovisual—information on audiovisual materials, in published or unpublished form; dial-access—telephone access to tapes or knowledgeable persons; research projects information sources—provide published or unpublished information on current projects; registries—maintain and provide epidemiological data; organizations—sponsor/meetings and/or provide grants; National Institutes of Health programs and services—Government programs or publications. *The Audiovisual Information Sources Section* is divided into four areas: comprehensive sources, motion pictures, videotapes, audio-filmstrips, visual materials: slides, filmstrips, overhead transparencies, and audio materials, which cover the following specific subject areas: abstracts, bibliographies, community health, computers (information systems), dentistry, documents, educa-

tion, medicine (under specific topics), neoplasms, nursing, organizations, preventive medicine, public health (information to the public), research, resources, and safety.

ENTRIES Title, publisher's address and phone number, country of publication, name to contact, scope of publication, topics included, description of entries, cataloging information, audience, ordering information, price.

SPECIAL FEATURES Includes title, organization, geographic and subject indexes, and gives information on the activities of the national and international agencies which cooperate in the ICRDB Program.

ORDERING INFORMATION Available from the NTIS Rept. No.: NCI/ICRDB/DI-77/01.

PRICE $3.50.

DISASTER PREPAREDNESS: PUBLICATIONS, FILMS, and OTHER AUDIO-VISUAL MATERIALS from the NATIONAL WEATHER SERVICE

National Oceanic and Atmospheric Administration. U.S. Department of Commerce. [1980]. [8] p.

MEDIA	16mm films, slide sets.
SUMMARY	This brochure includes both print and nonprint materials dealing with all aspects of natural disasters. Publications are available at a nominal cost from the National Oceanic and Atmospheric Administration, while the 31 nonprint media are available from the National Audiovisual Center for rental or purchase. Some audiovisuals are available in Spanish.
ENTRIES	Title, running time, markings for physical description, format, annotation.
SPECIAL FEATURES	Includes print materials related to audiovisual materials. Ordering information is also included. Some audiovisuals are also available in Spanish.
ORDERING INFORMATION	Available from the Superintendent of Documents, U.S. Government Printing Office: NOAA/PA 76021 (Rev. June 1980).
PRICE	$1.50. Single copy free from the National Oceanic and Atmospheric Administration.

DOCUMENTARY FILM CLASSICS PRODUCED by the UNITED STATES GOVERNMENT

National Audiovisual Center, National Archives and Records Service. U.S. General Services Administration. 1980. 48 p. Plus announcements.

MEDIA	16mm films.
SUMMARY	This "special issue" includes some of the finest documentaries ever made all produced by the U.S. Government since the 1930's. They depict the growing pains of wars, ecology, exploitation and misuse of the environment, development of community medical care, the struggle of immigrant workers for food and health, hospital work in prisons, occupational health, use of psychology during war, social problems in a segregated society, and the roots of the Vietnam war. These films have been shown all over the world and have received numerous honors and awards including Academy Awards. The names associated with their production are: Frank Capra, Henri Cartier-Bresson, Robert Flaherty, John Ford, John Huston, Joris Ivens, Garson Kanin, Pare Lorentz, Carol Reed, Willard Van Dyke, Josel von Stemberg, William Wyler, and other artists such as Toscanini, Copland, Steinbeck, Gruenberg and many TV and Motion Picture personalities. Through this catalog, The National Audiovisual Center extends the services of the National Archives and Records Services by making these films more widely available. All films listed in the catalog are complete versions reproduced from the original print and nonprint materials.
ENTRIES	Title, running time, color or b/w, year of release, credits, annotation, comments on theme, setting and content, review(s), format, film number, availability, rental and purchase price, award(s). A picture and the name of producer(s) are accompanying each film.
SPECIAL FEATURES	Includes notes from the National Audiovisual Center, bibliography of print materials related to the films, purchase and rental policies, and a title index.
ORDERING INFORMATION	Available from The National Audiovisual Center.
PRICE	Free.

DRUG ABUSE FILMS. Compiled by Richard W. Sackett

Office of Communications and Public Affairs, National Institutes on Drug Abuse, Public Health Service, Alcohol, Drug Abuse, and Mental Health Administration. U.S. Department of Health, Education, and Welfare. 1980. 26 p.

MEDIA	16mm films.
SUMMARY	This catalog includes 61 drug abuse films which have been released during the past ten years and which aim at the audiences most frequently mentioned by requesters. The list includes films both privately and federally produced. These films are currently available from their distributors for sale, rent, or on a free loan basis. Topics included are: community and drug use, counseling and crisis intervention, drug education and education in general, drugs and their effects, family life and drug use, imprisonment, law enforcement, legal aspects of drug use, medical and pharmacological aspects of drug use, pharmacology, prevention, teacher training in drug education, treatment facilities and techniques, and treatment and rehabilitation.
ENTRIES	Title, year of release/production, name and address of distributor, running time, sale price and/or information on rental and loan, policies, target audience, and annotation.
SPECIAL FEATURES	Provides a list of other federal sources of information, topical index, section on new films, and audience index.
ORDERING INFORMATION	Available from the Superintendent of Documents, U.S. Government Printing Office: 1980—311-246-6014. DHEW Publication No. (ADM) 80-914.
PRICE	Single copy available free of charge from the Office of Communications and Public Affairs, National Institutes on Drug Abuse.

DRUG ABUSE PREVENTION FILMS: A MULTICULTURAL FILM CATALOG

National Institute on Drug Abuse, Division of Resource Development, Prevention Branch. Alcohol, Drug Abuse, and Mental Health Administration. U.S. Department of Health, Education, and Welfare. 1978. 52 p.

(This publication was prepared for the National Institute of Resource and Development, Prevention Branch, Center for Multicultural Awareness, under Contract No. 271-77-4525 to Develop Associates, Inc., Arlington, Virginia.)

MEDIA	16mm films.
SUMMARY	About 150 current films produced by both U.S. Government agencies and independent producers, are described in this catalog. They cover drug abuse prevention topics centering on five minority groups: Asian/Pacific Islanders, Blacks, Mexican Americans, Puerto Ricans, and Native Americans. These materials can be used in drug programs, community centers, schools, libraries, and by groups concerned about the primary prevention of drug abuse within minority groups. They portray young people growing up and making choices about their lives within the context of their cultural and ethnic background, and social environment. The catalog is divided into the following sections: recommended films (films reviewed by members of the Center for Multicultural Awareness (CMA) staff, and others, and found to be particularly useful to minority prevention programs and to be of good technical quality; other films reviewed (films reviewed by the CMA) but were found to be inappropriate for primary prevention programs for minorities; other sources of film reviews and evaluations; and subject index to useful films section which is organized by subject matter of films: Asian/Pacific Islander, Black, Mexican American, Puerto Rican, multicultural, films in Spanish, drugs, personal values, cultural values, cross cultural, life skills, alternatives, parent education, and staff training. Many films are in Spanish.
ENTRIES	Title, distributor, color or b/w, format, running time, rental or purchase price, year of release, cross reference, audience level, annotation, films reviewed.
SPECIAL FEATURES	Includes notes on reviewed items, reviewer, information on other films reviewed but not included in the catalog (their content not appropriate for minorities), and other films (which are often free of charge), evaluations, distributors list, forms for audience comments. A subject index for useful films is also included.

ORDERING INFORMATION Available from the National Institute on Drug Abuse, Division of Resource Development, Prevention Branch, Center for Multicultural Awareness. DHEW Publication No. (ADM) 79-791. U.S. Government Printing Office: 1978:-281-265/1220. Also available from NTIS.

PRICE Single copy free from The National Institute on Drug Abuse. NTIS price not available. Also available from ERIC in microfiche.

EDUCATIONAL MEDIA RESOURCES on EGYPT

Office of Education. U.S. Department of Health, Education, and Welfare. 1977. 57 p.

(This directory was prepared by the University of Michigan, Audio-Visual Education Center, Ann Arbor, pursuant to a contract with the Office of Education, U.S. Department of Health, Education, and Welfare.)

MEDIA	8mm, 16mm, 35mm films, filmstrips, videocassettes, slide sets, audiotapes, kits, recordings.
SUMMARY	This directory includes 424 audiovisual entries produced by independent producers, colleges and universities, associations, including the United Nations, since 1950. These audiovisuals deal mostly with the history of Egypt's civilization including agriculture, archeology, geography, language and literature on Mediterranean countries and their civilization, political, social and technological problems, and transportation. Broad health sciences subjects included are: animal life, climatology, energy (natural resources), environment, infant mortality, irrigation, medical education, natural disasters, sciences (general), and thanatology. The life and work of Dr. David Livingston is also included in these films. Many motion picture personalities serve as narrators in many films.
ENTRIES	Title, captions (when appropriate), accompanying print material, running time or number of frames, sound or silent, color or b/w, audience level, annotation, producer/distributor, year of release.
SPECIAL FEATURES	Includes introduction explaining the cooperation between the Office of Education and the Joint Cooperation Commission on Education and Culture. A list of distributors and subject index are also included.
ORDERING INFORMATION	Available from the Superintendent of Documents, U.S. Government Printing Office: 177 0-245-499. Stock No. 017-080-01789-0.
PRICE	$1.50.

ENERGY EFFICIENCY SHARING: BUSINESS-to-BUSINESS PROGRAM to FACILITATE EXCHANGE of ENERGY MANAGEMENT TECHNOLOGY and TECHNIQUES

National Industrial Council, Office of Field Operations, Office of Energy Programs. U.S. Department of Domestic and International Business Administration. February 1977. [8] p. Plus announcements.

MEDIA	16mm films.
SUMMARY	This brochure includes a list of U.S. Government publications and films on energy. This particular issue (February 1977) includes a 16mm, 18-minute film entitled "Energy: Critical Choices Ahead" which can be borrowed from the U.S. Department of Commerce District Office or purchased from the Office of Energy Programs, U.S. Department of Commerce. Those interested in additional later productions, should place their names on the mailing list for future publications and announcements.
ENTRIES	Descriptions of single films appear as a footnote under the section "U.S. Government Publications and Films." Gives title, format, running time, availability. For more information write to U.S. Department of Commerce District Office or Office of Energy Programs, U.S. Department of Commerce, Washington, D.C. 20230.
SPECIAL FEATURES	This brochure is published on an irregular basis to inform the public about the cooperation of major U.S. corporations with the U.S. Department of Commerce and the Federal Energy Administration (FEA) on the Energy Efficiency Sharing Programs. It includes a list of publications published by the Department of Commerce, including audiovisuals.
ORDERING INFORMATION	Available from the Superintendent of Documents, U.S. Government Printing Office.
PRICE	35 cents. Single copy free from U.S. Department of Commerce, Washington, D.C. 20230.

ENERGY FILMS CATALOG

Audiovisual Branch, Office of Public Affairs. Energy Research and Development Administration. 1976. 71 p. Plus supplements.

(For films available from the U.S. Department of Energy see "35 Energy Films" catalog included in this book. Full library audiovisual services from the Oak Ridge National Laboratory temporarily suspended.)

MEDIA	16mm films.
SUMMARY	Includes 188 films produced by both U.S. Government agencies and independent producers for the Energy Research and Development Administration (ERDA). The collection represents many of the energy options offered by ERDA and its related activities. All are designed for schools, television stations, civic clubs, government and industrial organizations interested in educational and informational films as well as technical and professional films on energy and energy related subjects on three levels: elementary, high school, and college and university; industry, researchers, scientists; engineers and technologists. The catalog is arranged in six major divisions: solar, geothermal and advanced energy systems, nuclear energy, energy conservation, environment and safety, and national security. Subjects included in the six broad categories are: accelerator, agriculture, anthropology, atomic elements, atomic energy, atomic (nuclear) power, biology, breeder reactor, careers, challenge series, computers, conservation, controlled thermonuclear reactor, cyclotron, data processing, electricity, energy, energy centers, engineering, environment, fossil, fusion, geothermal, medicine, metallurgy, national laboratories energy centers, national security, nuclear power, peaceful nuclear explosives, personalities, physics, radiation, radioisotopes, research, research and test reactors, safeguards, safety, solar energy, space, SNAP (Systems for Nuclear Auxiliary Power), transportation, understanding the atom series. The films have received numerous national and international awards and are available to the public on a free-loan basis. Color stock footage of these films is available (under special agreement) to producers.
ENTRIES	Film number, title, running time, color or b/w, series, audience, TV clearance, annotation, honors and awards.
SPECIAL FEATURES	Includes information on how to obtain films for viewing, footage, or duplication, subject and title indexes, listing of sponsors, sales sources, and film order forms.

ORDERING INFORMATION Available from the Energy Research and Development Administration and U.S. Government Printing Office: 1976-647-617.

PRICE Single copy free.

ENGINEERING: SELECTED U.S. GOVERNMENT AUDIOVISUALS

National Audiovisual Center, National Archives and Records Service. U.S. General Services Administration. June 1977. 44 p.

MEDIA	16mm films, filmstrips, videocassettes, slide sets, audiocassettes, transparencies.
SUMMARY	About 150 audiovisual materials are described in this catalog which are produced by the U.S. Government dealing with civil, mechanical, general, nuclear, environmental, marine, and industrial engineering. Specific subjects covered are: atomic power safety, construction safety on national and international levels, energy, environmental engineering, hazardous waste, industrial safety, noise, ocean instrumentation/submarine, pollution, submarine safety, recycling, sanitation, space technology, terradynamics. Most of these materials are current but some of them date back to 1950.
ENTRIES	Title, running time or number of frames, format, sound or silent, color or b/w, year of release, producer, title number, sale price, annotation, TV clearance, language (if other than English).
SPECIAL FEATURES	Gives information on other catalogs published by the National Audiovisual Center, ordering information, information on public services by the Center. Title index is also included.
ORDERING INFORMATION	Available from The National Audiovisual Center.
PRICE	Free.

ENVIRONMENTAL MOVIES and SLIDE SHOWS from EPA

United States Environmental Protection Agency. Office of Public Awareness. December 1980. 12 p. Plus announcements.

MEDIA	16mm films, slide sets.
SUMMARY	The 30 current audiovisual entries produced by the U.S. Environmental Protection Agency represent the Agency's integrated attack on environmental protection in cooperation with state and local agencies. They also show how national and environmental laws, which protect the Nation's land, air, and water systems mandate by Congress, are reinforced. The audiovisuals in which many TV, motion pictures, sports, and music personalities from U.S. and Canada appear, have received national and international awards and are available to the public on a free-loan basis through the National Audiovisual Center or EPA offices around the country. Some entries are available in Spanish.
ENTRIES	Title, running time or number of frames, year of release, format, sound or silent, b/w, annotation, distributing offices.
SPECIAL FEATURES	Includes pertinent information on the activities of EPA, name and addresses of distributing agencies and offices, and EPA relation to the U.S. Congress.
ORDERING INFORMATION	Available from the Environmental Protection Agency.
PRICE	Free.

FAA FILM CATALOG [for Public Use]

Federal Aviation Administration. U.S. Department of Transportation. 1976. 20 p.

MEDIA	16mm, filmstrips, audioslide sets.
SUMMARY	Includes 230 audiovisuals produced and distributed by the Federal Aviation Administration through the Administration's Regional Offices. Each film is a documentary and provides information on the following broad subjects: aerodynamics and flight conditions, aircraft safety, airports, aviation history (beginning with the Wright Brothers), aviation medicine, crash and fire rescue, general aviation and flying clubs (educational), inspection and maintenance, international aviation, navigation, research and development, weather (air masses and fronts, atmospheric conditions), and general metereology. Most of the programs have received national and international awards.
ENTRIES	Title, annotation, running time, year of release, FAA ordering film number, purchase price.
SPECIAL FEATURES	Includes an introduction explaining the content of the films in relation to the Federal Aviation Administration, general information to the users, and information on television showing restrictions, rental and purchase details. Subject index and graphic information of FAA Regional Public Affairs Offices are also included.
ORDERING INFORMATION	Available from the Superintendent of Documents, U.S. Government Printing Office: 1974 0-537-880.
PRICE	$2.95. Free copy from the Federal Aviation Administration.

FEDERAL EMERGENCY MANAGEMENT AGENCY MOTION PICTURE CATALOG

Federal Emergency Management Agency. June 1980. 33 p.

MEDIA	16mm films.
SUMMARY	This catalog includes 40 current films produced by the Federal Emergency Management designed for training and orientation, and to bring information to the public in order to promote more effective emergency management. Subjects included are: aerospace sciences, emergency preparedness efforts of the United States in industry, environmental sciences, first aid, geology, natural disasters, nuclear fallout protection and management, public safety, safety/engineering/physics/earthquakes, and rescue missions. The films which have received numerous national and international awards are available in the U.S. and abroad on a free-loan basis from the nearest Army Training & Audiovisual Support Centers (TASC) listed in this catalog, or in foreign countries, through the U.S. Embassy or Consulate in the country concerned. Film footage of the FEMA films is also available under certain conditions, or transfered to ¾" videocassette format under agreement with the Agency.
ENTRIES	Title, running time, color or b/w, annotation, TV clearance, date of release, availability.
SPECIAL FEATURES	Includes general information on the activities of the agency, instruction for requesting motion pictures from U.S. and foreign countries, information for purchase and availability in general, alphabetical index, a list of obsolete motion pictures, addresses of major Army Training and Audiovisual Support Centers by State and Territories, order form for film loans, and a list of other subject related catalogs available from other agencies.
ORDERING INFORMATION	Available from the Federal Emergency Management Agency.
PRICE	Free.

FILM ARCHIVES on CHILD DEVELOPMENT—The INAUGURATION of the CHILD DEVELOPMENT ARCHIVES

Sponsored in part by the Office of Human Development. U.S. Department of Health, Education, and Welfare. Contract No. 90-C984. Final Report—December 19, 1978. 9 p. [Popplestone, John A. and Marion White McPherson]

MEDIA	8mm, 16mm, 32mm films, filmstrips.
SUMMARY	This cataloging of films acquired by the Child Development Film Archives consists of approximately 4,000 films donated by the following individuals and organizations:

Originals	Donor	Films
Arnold Gesell	Yale University	2,048
L. Joseph Stone	L.J. Stone and Vassar College	1,048
Margaret Mahler	M. Mahler	264
Miscellaneous	Various Individuals	15
	Total	3,491

Each film is accompanied by an inventory sheet which provides a record of the content of each cinema (film). Variables specified on inventory sheets include: children—number, sex, age, ethnicity, amount and nature of clothing, biopathology, and psychopathology. Adults—number, sex, and interaction with children. Animals—number and species. For each category there is an enumeration of the specific activities depicted. The milieu in which the action occurs is identified. Changes in content within a film are recorded and the resulting variations in subjects are noted. Identifying data also included on existence and location of relevant documents. NOTE: The collection is currently housed in Bierce Library at the University of Akron, Ohio.

ENTRIES	Title, purpose, sound or silent, relevant existing documents, color or b/w, notes regarding visual (and audio) clarity, cast/credits, length of footage, width, running time, identification number of item, storage location, availability.
SPECIAL FEATURES	Includes the Gesell early studies on child psychology.
ORDERING INFORMATION	Available from National Technical Information Service. Is also available from ERIC Document Reproduction on Microfiche.
PRICE	$4.95.

FILM CATALOG

U.S. Fish and Wildlife Service. U.S. Department of the Interior. [1979]. [9] p.

MEDIA	16mm films.
SUMMARY	This catalog includes 65 films concerning fish and wildlife sciences. These films are available on a free-loan basis to schools, groups, clubs, organizations, and individuals interested in the history and preservation of fish and wildlife. Subjects covered by the films are: animal and wildlife in general, animal preservation, animal reproduction, bionomics, ecological evolution, energy and conservation, environmental sciences, food, geology, lake and river restoration, marine biology, marine life, natural resources, pesticides/effects on animal life and nature, physiological adaptation of animals, the history of the U.S. Fish and Wildlife Services and its activities depicting the need to strike a balance between man and nature, water pollution, weather, and Mutual of Omaha's series on wildlife presentations. The films, in which many motion pictures and TV personalities appear, have received many awards.
ENTRIES	Title, audience, running time, annotation, awards, (n.d.).
SPECIAL FEATURES	Includes information on other sources of free film services, loan information, and policies.
ORDERING INFORMATION	Available from the U.S. Department of the Interior, Fish and Wildlife Services.
PRICE	Free.

FILM FARE: A CATALOG of FILMS and FILMSTRIPS PRODUCED by the U.S. DEPARTMENT of HOUSING and URBAN DEVELOPMENT.

U.S. Department of Housing and Urban Development, Office of Public Affairs. September [1974]. [11] p.

MEDIA	16mm films, filmstrips.
SUMMARY	This catalog includes 24 audiovisual presentations produced since 1967 covering the following subject areas: architecture, environment, housing crisis, HUD's involvement in urban housing, neighborhoods for senior citizens' activities, nursing homes, pollution, recreation, transportation, and urban renewal. Materials are available on a free-loan basis from the twenty-seven libraries of Modern Talking Pictures, Inc. or HUD's Regional Offices listed in this catalog.
ENTRIES	Title, annotation, format, running time, availability, year of release, producer, distributor.
SPECIAL FEATURES	Includes a list of Modern Talking Picture Services, a list of Regional and Area Offices of the Department of Housing and Urban Development (HUD), pictures accompanying entries, and subject index.
ORDERING INFORMATION	Available from the U.S. Department of Housing and Urban Development, HUD: 192-PA (2).
PRICE	Free.

FILM GUIDE on REPRODUCTION and DEVELOPMENT: *A Guide to Selected Films on Reproductive and Developmental Biology for Graduate and Undergraduate Programs in the Biomedical Sciences*

National Institutes of Health, Public Health Service. U.S. Department of Health, Education, and Welfare. [1970]. 66 p.

(Prepared by the National Institute of Child Health and Human Development.)

MEDIA	16mm films.
SUMMARY	The 26 films included in this guide have been selected for their usefulness and appropriateness in educational settings ranging from the undergraduate level on through graduate schools concerned with professional education. The major area of interest in these films demonstrates the fundamental process of reproduction. Specific subjects covered are: structure and function of cells, mitosis and meiosis, development of invertebrata/osteichthyes/amphibia, differentiation and organogenesis, courtship and reproduction, laboratory techniques. The guide contains highly specialized and unusual materials such as the film "Triturus Taeniatus (Salamandridae) ZWILLINGSBILDUNG Twin Formation in the Salamander" (produced in the Institut fur den Wissenschaftlichen Film), where time-lapse cinematography illustrates the synchrony of early cell division in the two eggs followed by scenes of neurulation, and twinning is produced by separating the blastomeres in the two-cell stage with a loop of very fine hair, while in another experiment the ventral half of the fertilized egg is partially separated from the dorsal half by the hair-loop.
ENTRIES	Title, format, sound or silent, color or b/w, running time, number of reels, author(s) and his/their affiliation, target audience, annotation, references (citations), distributor(s), accompanying materials, rental and purchase prices, related notes.
SPECIAL FEATURES	Includes a subject index under the table of contents and ordering instructions.
ORDERING INFORMATION	Superintendent of Documents, U.S. Government Printing Office: 1970-352-815.
PRICE	[$1.25] (temporarily o.p.).

FILM RESOURCES on JAPAN

Office of Education. U.S. Department of Health, Education, and Welfare. 1975. 55 p.

(This directory was prepared by the University of Michigan, Audio-Visual Educational Center, Ann Arbor, pursuant to a contract with the Office of Education, U.S. Department of Health, Education, and Welfare.)

MEDIA	16mm films, filmstrips.
SUMMARY	This catalog includes 500 audiovisual entries produced by commercial producers, colleges and universities, associations including the United Nations. These audiovisuals deal primarily with the history of Japanese civilization, agriculture, archeology, geography, language, literature, political and social problems, and technology. It also includes the following health sciences area subjects: animal life, atomic energy, climatology, education, effects of the atomic bomb on humans (the Hiroshima incident), energy, environmental sciences, family life, food and nutrition, natural resources, recreation, safety, sociology, transportation, urbanization. These materials have been produced since 1960. A list of films produced prior to that year are listed in a separate section.
ENTRIES	Title, running time, format, color or b/w, audience level, annotation, producer and distributor, year of release.
SPECIAL FEATURES	Includes introduction explaining the cooperation between the Office of Education and the Joint Committee on Culture and Educational Cooperation, separate section of films produced before 1960, sponsored films (free loan), a list of 35mm films, distributors list, and subject index.
ORDERING INFORMATION	Available from the Superintendent of Documents, U.S. Government Printing Office.
PRICE	$1.50.

FILMS: FREE from the NATIONAL BUREAU of STANDARDS

National Bureau of Standards. U.S. Department of Commerce. [September, 1978]. 20 p.

MEDIA	16mm films, videocassettes.
SUMMARY	Includes 34 audiovisual entries produced by the U.S. National Bureau of Standards. These films are previewed by the NBS researchers and are available on a free-loan basis to scientific and professional organizations, educational institutions, and nonprofit community organizations. Although some films are over 40 years old, the information they present is still accurate and useful for the target audience. The catalog is divided in three sections: 1) general science, 2) technical, and 3) dental, and includes the following broad subject categories: casting (dental), chemistry, computers (industrial), consumer information in the marketplace, difractometer control system, electronic technology, engineering, fire safety, law enforcement equipment standards, lead and paint poisoning, measures of air quality, noise control, radiation (oral), safety devices, spectographic radiation, thermodynamics, toys, household products and house designing safety.
ENTRIES	Title, format, running time, year of release, annotation, audience level, subject(s), co-producer.
SPECIAL FEATURES	Includes a map of the Association Films Distribution Centers, ordering information, and film loan agreement form/request.
ORDERING INFORMATION	Available from the National Bureau of Standards, U.S. Department of Commerce.
PRICE	Free.

FOREST SERVICE FILMS AVAILABLE on LOAN to the PUBLIC for EDUCATIONAL PURPOSES

U.S. Forest Service. Eastern Region (Milwaukee, Wis.). U.S. Department of Agriculture. 1979. 15 p.

MEDIA	16mm films, filmstrips.
SUMMARY	Includes 194 audiovisuals covering the following subject areas: agriculture, animals and wildlife, environmental issues, fire safety and fire prevention, flood control, food packaging, forestry, gardening, irrigation, natural resources, recreation, and sports. Most items are current, although some materials included have been produced as early as 1948. NOTE: Some entries are included in the Pacific Northern Region catalog.
ENTRIES	Title, running time, color or b/w, grade level, annotation, film library number, TV clearance.
SPECIAL FEATURES	Gives a list of States served by this Region.
ORDERING INFORMATION	Available from the Forest Service, U.S. Department of Agriculture, Eastern Region Information Office.
PRICE	Free.

A GUIDE TO AUDIO-VISUAL AIDS for COURSES in the HISTORY of LATIN AMERICAN CIVILIZATION in HIGHER EDUCATION INSTITUTIONS

National Institute of Education, Bureau of Research, Office of Education. U.S. Department of Health, Education, and Welfare. Regional Research Program. Boston, January 1973. 100 p.

(This report was prepared by the National Institute of Education, Regional Research Program, Boston, Project No. IA057 under a grant from the U.S. Department of Health, Education, and Welfare. Grant No. CEG-1-72-0002(509).

MEDIA	16mm films.
SUMMARY	Sixty-four educational and 13 feature evaluated films are described in this report, dealing with the following Latin American countries: Argentina, Brazil, Bolivia, Central America, Chile, Columbia, Cuba, Dominican Republic, Equador, Mexico, and Venezuela. These films are produced by both U.S. Government agencies and independent producers in U.S. and Canada since 1940, covering the following subject areas: agriculture, anthropology, archeology, bionomics, geography, life in the Amazon, Peruvian Indian life, population explosion, sociology, urbanization.
ENTRIES	Title, b/w, running time, producer, series, year of release, distributor(s), rental and purchase price, annotation, appraisal, evaluation, suggested readings (bibliographies), audience.
SPECIAL FEATURES	Includes sections on recommended educational and feature films, ordering information, title index, supplementary readings.
ORDERING INFORMATION	Available from ERIC Documents Reproduction Service.
PRICE	$4.50.

GUIDE to AUDIOVISUAL AIDS for SPANISH-SPEAKING AMERICANS

Health Services Administration, Public Health Service. U.S. Department of Health, Education, and Welfare. 1973. 37 p.

MEDIA	16mm films, filmstrips, slide sets.
SUMMARY	This catalog is a guide to all health workers on communications aids which are particularly suited for use with Spanish-speaking Americans. Many of these audiovisuals have received national and international awards. Includes 250 audiovisuals classified under 26 subject areas: accident prevention and occupational health, aging, community health, dental health, diseases and conditions (cancer, colds, diabetes, emphysema, heart disease, including rheumatic fever and high blood pressure and its treatment, mental retardation, multiple sclerosis, tuberculosis, venereal disease), emergency health care, family planning, the human body and its development, mental health (alcoholism and alcohol abuse, drug abuse), migrant health, nutrition and food sanitation, personal hygiene, physical fitness, prenatal and infant care, smoking and health. Some of the materials cited may be available on a free-loan basis or rental from local sources such as public libraries, health and welfare agencies, film libraries, and schools.
ENTRIES	Title, format, sound or silent, color or b/w, running time or number of frames, year of release, rental or purchase price, annotation, audience level, awards.
SPECIAL FEATURES	Includes distributors list. Many Walt Disney films are also included.
ORDERING INFORMATION	Available from the Department of Health, Education, and Welfare, DHEW Publication No. (HSA) 74-30.
PRICE	Single copy free.

HEALTH, 1980-81

National Audiovisual Center, National Archives and Records Service. U.S. General Services Administration. [1981]. 24 p.

MEDIA	16mm films, videocassettes, slide sets.
SUMMARY	This catalog includes approximately 100 audiovisuals recently produced by the U.S. Government. These audiovisuals are designed to help consumers expand their knowledge about their own health care, and how their bodies are affected by life style and environment. Topics included are: child abuse, Walt Disney Classics (cartoon characters spotlight historical health perspectives), drug abuse/alcohol abuse, first aid, physical fitness, from pregnancy to parenthood (depicting the challenges and changes that the child brings), Health Care Organization (series), the health professional, nutrition, occupational health, patient education. A series of "medicine for the laymen" is also included. Some entries are available in Spanish. The audiovisual materials have received numerous awards.
ENTRIES	Title, annotation, award(s), running time or number of frames, year of release, accompanying print material(s), producing agency, format, film number, rental and sales information, availability in other format(s), awards.
ORDERING INFORMATION	Available from The National Audiovisual Center.
PRICE	Free.

IN FOCUS: ALCOHOL and ALCOHOLISM MEDIA

National Clearinghouse for Alcohol Information, National Institute on Alcohol Abuse and Alcoholism, Alcohol, Drug Abuse and Mental Health Administration, Public Health Service. U.S. Department of Health, Education, and Welfare. 1980. 86 p.

MEDIA	16mm films, filmstrips, videocassettes, slide sets, audiocassettes.
SUMMARY	This catalog is published by the National Clearinghouse for Alcohol Information of the National Institute on Alcohol and Alcoholism as a review of materials currently available on alcohol abuse and alcoholism. Includes 300 audiovisuals produced since 1960, but also includes some produced since 1950, for both the scientific and professional community as well as the general public. Subjects covered are: abstinence, acupuncture, alcohol beverage industry, alcohol/drug interaction, Alcoholics Anonymous, alcohol safety action projects, alternatives, American Indians, attitudes, aviation, behavior, blacks, case histories, criminal offenses, dependence and withdrawal syndromes, drinking habits/cultural, drug abuse, education, emergencies, etiology, foreign language, Halfway Houses, history of alcohol use, hospital programs, hotlines, media campaigns, men, minorities, nutrition, occupational alcoholism, physiology, prevention, psychology of drinking, rehabilitation and treatment, smoking, social problems, therapy, women, youth. Some programs present problems of addiction which occur in Russian, Spanish, and French cultures. New audiovisuals appear in the *niaaa information and feature service*. (A Newsletter available from the National Clearinghouse.)
ENTRIES	Title, format, year of release, running time, color or b/w, TV clearance, language (of other than English), source, audience level, sale and rental information, distributor, annotation, awards.
SPECIAL FEATURES	Includes a list of publications relating to media resources, a list of information centers to call for help, and subject and title indexes. TV clearance information is also included. Awards.
ORDERING INFORMATION	Available from the Superintendent of Documents, U.S. Government Printing Office: 1980-311.246.6116. DHEW Publication No. (ADM) 80-32.
PRICE	$1.50.

INDEX of ARMY MOTION PICTURES for PUBLIC NON-PROFIT USE

U.S. Department of the Army Headquarters. Washington, D.C. February 1980. 60 p.

MEDIA	16mm films.
SUMMARY	This U.S. Army Pamphlet includes approximately 1,000 films produced by the United States Army or for the Army by other Government agencies since 1940. These are available to government, civic, religious, fraternal and educational groups, schools, colleges, universities, and other agencies interested in non-profit showings of Army films to the general public. Many films are classified as "historical" and are still available for viewing. Entries are grouped under the following categories: Armed Forces information films, Army information films, combat miscellaneous films, defense civil preparedness films, information and educational sports reels, professional medical films, recruiting films, TV: Television "Big Picture" films. Health sciences broad subject areas covered throughout these categories are: animal laboratory research, atomic medical cases, aviation, death, defense civil preparedness, dermatology, dentistry, drug detection, environmental sciences, heat stroke, hematology, medical teamwork in Vietnam, nursing, oral hygiene, osteopathy, physical therapy, psychology (propaganda), radiology, research and development, tropical diseases, work of the U.S. Army Environmental Hygiene Agency in Vietnam on pesticide control.
SPECIAL FEATURES	Includes sections on purpose and scope of the films, procedures for ordering films, areas of service (procurement), Army Training and Audiovisual Centers (by State), use of films, purchase of the Department of the Army films, and reference materials available from the Army Film Distribution Department.
ORDERING INFORMATION	Available from the Superintendent of Documents, U.S. Government Printing Office: Department of the Army Pamphlet No. 180-4. 1980-603-128/1422.
PRICE	Free.

INDIANS in the UNITED STATES: SELECT AUDIOVISUAL RECORDS

The National Archives Trust Fund Board. U.S. General Services Administration. 1975. 18 p.

MEDIA	Still photographs.
SUMMARY	The pictures listed in this brochure portray American Indians, their homes and activities. They have been selected from pictorial records deposited in the National Archives by 15 Government agencies, principally the Bureau of Indian Affairs, the Bureau of American Ethnology, and the U.S. Army. The audiovisuals are arranged under 24 broad categories representing the following subjects: agriculture, anthropology, child rearing and education, fishery, food preparation, hunting, men (religion), prison life, transportation, war/army sciences (includes WW II), and women (religion). NOTE: There are many other audiovisuals relating to North American Indians in the Audiovisual Archives, the Division of the National Archives and the Bureau of Indian Affairs, Department of the Interior, Washington, D.C. 20240. To request a picture not included in this brochure, a form request is included with directions on how the request should be made.
ENTRIES	Number of item, name (of specific person or a tribe), length, position of portrait (when applicable), photographer, date, order number (more specific).
SPECIAL FEATURES	Includes a list/index of 65 tribes, each tribe accompanied by a number for ordering purpose, and an order form.
ORDERING INFORMATION	Available from the Superintendent of Documents, U.S. Government Printing Office Stock Number 022-000-00094-2.
PRICE	40 cents.

LIBROS PARLANTES (Talking Book Topics)

Publication Services, Division for the Blind and Physically Handicapped. U.S. Library of Congress. 1972-. (Three Spanish Language Catalogs.) [1980, 3rd ed.]

MEDIA	Cassettes.
SUMMARY	This publication includes 117 titles recorded in Spanish for the national talking-book program from 1973 through 1980. Most of the titles are talking-book cassettes, in keeping with the policy to record all new Spanish titles in cassettes. (See TALKING BOOK TOPICS for subjects). *(See also Catalog of Educational Films for the Deaf 1980-81.)*
ENTRIES	Title, author, narrator(s), identification number, annotation, year of publication.
SPECIAL FEATURES	Includes information on how to use the system, eligibility, ordering information, surveys and studies, and related print materials. Subscription and order forms are also included.
PRICE	Free copies of this publication is available at cooperating public libraries.

LIBRARY of CONGRESS CATALOGS: AUDIOVISUAL MATERIALS 1980*
(Formerly FILMS and OTHER MATERIALS for PROJECTION 1973-1979)

U.S. Library of Congress. 1981. (Quarterly [January-March, April-June, July-September], with annual and quinquennial cumulations.)

MEDIA	16mm films, filmstrips, videocassettes, slide sets, kits, transparencies, recordings.
SUMMARY	This catalog includes approximately 15,000 audiovisuals currently catalogued by the U.S. Library of Congress. It is comprehensive in scope in that it includes all educational and instructional audiovisuals released in the United States and Canada for which the Library of Congress prints Library of Congress catalog cards. These cards represent audiovisuals cataloged by the Library of Congress and by libraries and institutions contributing to its cooperative cataloging program. Data for this catalog is supplied by producers, manufacturers, film libraries, or distributing agencies. Information for audiovisuals produced by the U.S. Government is provided by the National Audiovisual Center. Broad subject categories in medicine and allied health sciences include: abortion, aged, accidents, aeronautics, agriculture, alcohol and alcoholism, anesthesiology, arthritis, audiometry, behavioral sciences (animals and humans), biology, blood, bones, cancer, cardiovascular system, chemistry, child abuse, communicable diseases, cytology, dentistry, drugs and drug abuse, ecology, education (medical, special), electronics (medical), embryology, emergency, endocrine system, energy, environment, epidemiology, first aid in illness and injury, food and nutrition, halfway houses, handicapped, human ecology, human reproduction, hypertension, industrial medicine, marine biology, medical ethics, medical jurisprudence, mental hygiene, musculoskeletal system, nursing, otorhinolaryngology, pediatrics, physical fitness, psychology and psychiatry, rehabilitation, safety, sex (education), skin, social sciences, surgery, technology (agriculture, industry, food), veterinary medicine, WHO (the work of the Pan American Health Organization), zoology. A subject index is provided based on *Subject Headings Used in Dictionary Catalogs of the Library of Congress.*
ENTRIES	Title, format, producer/distributor, year of release, running time or number of frames, sound or silent, color or b/w, credits, summary, subject(s), series, Library of Congress classification numbers, Dewey decimal classification number, Library of Congress card number, name of reporting (participating in the cataloging program) organization or institution.

SPECIAL FEATURES	It includes the history of the Library of Congress cataloging services (1951-), elements of entries, section, filing system information for catalogers, and a distributors list. Subject index is also included.
ORDERING INFORMATION	Available on subscription from the U.S. Library of Congress, Catalog Publication Division.
PRICE	$85.00. (3 quarterly issues and a case bound annual cumulation.)

A LIST of AUDIOVISUAL MATERIALS PRODUCED by the UNITED STATES GOVERNMENT for BUSINESS and GOVERNMENT MANAGEMENT

National Audiovisual Center, National Archives and Records Service. U.S. General Services Administration. 1980. 14 p.

MEDIA	16mm films, filmstrips, videocassettes, slide sets, audiotapes, multimedia kits.
SUMMARY	This directory contains 140 audiovisuals produced by the U.S. Government on management. Specific areas covered are: care of teeth and hair, skin, and good posture; a health maintenance organization as an alternative to health care delivery systems; providing quality health care; physicians' involvement in health care systems; selection and advancement of the handicapped, including training and environmental barriers. These audiovisuals are primarily intended for physicians who advise consumers, unions, and employers.
ENTRIES	Title, running time or number of frames, format, sound or silent, color or b/w, release date, producer, title number, sale price, annotation, TV clearance, language (if other than English).
SPECIAL FEATURES	Gives information on other catalogs published by the National Audiovisual Center, ordering information, and information on public services by the Center.
ORDERING INFORMATION	Available from The National Audiovisual Center.
PRICE	Free.

A LIST of AUDIOVISUAL MATERIALS PRODUCED by the UNITED STATES GOVERNMENT for CONSUMER EDUCATION

National Audiovisual Center, National Archives and Records Service. U.S. General Services Administration, 1980.

MEDIA	16mm films, filmstrips, videocassettes, slide sets, audiotapes, transparencies, multimedia kits.
SUMMARY	This directory contains 134 audiovisuals produced by the U.S. Government dealing with topics on consumer education. Specific subject areas include: consumer protection, dental health, driving safety (including court and trial procedures for driving under the influence of alcohol), emergency situations, injuries and death from accidents, housing and construction (including environmental barriers for handicapped persons), fire prevention and control, energy and conservation, and outdoor recreation. Some entries are in Spanish.
ENTRIES	Title, running time or number of frames, format, sound or silent, color or b/w, year of release, producer, title number, sale price, annotation, TV clearance, language (if other than English).
SPECIAL FEATURES	Gives information on other catalogs published by the National Audiovisual Center, ordering information, information on public services by the Center. Title index is also included.
ORDERING INFORMATION	Available from The National Audiovisual Center.
PRICE	Free.

A LIST of AUDIOVISUAL MATERIALS PRODUCED by the UNITED STATES GOVERNMENT for DRUG ABUSE PREVENTION

National Audiovisual Center, National Archives and Records Service, U.S. General Services Administration. [1980]. 13 p.

MEDIA	16mm films, filmstrips, videocassettes, slide sets, audiotapes, multimedia kits.
SUMMARY	This directory contains 123 audiovisuals produced by the U.S. Government dealing with alcohol and drug abuse prevention. Specific areas included are: alcohol and the body, alcohol and youth, alcohol counseling and rehabilitation, drugs and the body, drugs and youth, drug counseling and rehabilitation, and tobacco.
ENTRIES	Title, running time or number of frames, format, sound or silent, color or b/w, year of release, producer, title number, sale price, annotation, TV clearance, language (if other than English).
SPECIAL FEATURES	Gives information on other catalogs published by the National Audiovisual Center, ordering information, and information on public services by the Center. Title index is also included.
ORDERING INFORMATION	Available from the National Audiovisual Center.
PRICE	Free.

A LIST of AUDIOVISUAL MATERIALS PRODUCED by the UNITED STATES GOVERNMENT for EMERGENCY MEDICAL SERVICE

National Audiovisual Center, National Archives and Records Service, U.S. General Services Administration. [1980]. 11 p.

MEDIA	16mm films, filmstrips, videocassettes, slide sets, audiotapes, multimedia kits.
SUMMARY	Approximately 155 audiovisuals for both the layperson and the professional are included which cover all aspects of emergency medical services. Some of these areas are: civil defense, emergency childbirth, fallout, first aid, cardiopulmonary resuscitation (CPR), hurricane, instructor training series, military, physical fitness, physical shock, safety, and safety in schools. Some programs are in Spanish.
ENTRIES	Title, running time or number of frames, sound or silent, color or b/w, year of release, producer, title number, sale price, annotation, TV clearance, language (if other than English), audience level/for professional group or general public.
SPECIAL FEATURES	Gives information on other catalogs published by the National Audiovisual Center, title index, ordering information, and information on public services by the Center. Title index is also included.
ORDERING INFORMATION	Available from The National Audiovisual Center.
PRICE	Free.

A LIST of AUDIOVISUAL MATERIALS PRODUCED by the UNITED STATES GOVERNMENT for ENVIRONMENT and ENERGY CONSERVATION

National Audiovisual Center, National Archives and Records Service. U.S. General Services Administration. [1980]. 17 p.

MEDIA	16mm films, filmstrips, videocassettes, slide sets, audiotapes, multimedia kits.
SUMMARY	The 155 entries, all produced in 1971 or later, represent the following subject areas: air pollution, alternate energy sources, energy and energy conservation, general audiovisuals in environmental or energy conservation, land, noise, pollution, pesticides, solid waste, recycling, and waste. These materials are available for preview or purchase either from the National Audiovisual Center or the producing agencies.
ENTRIES	Title, running time or number of frames, format, sound or silent, color or b/w, year of release, producer, title number, sale price, annotation, TV clearance, language (if other than English).
SPECIAL FEATURES	Gives information on other catalogs published by the National Audiovisual Center, ordering information, information on public services by the Center. Title index is also included.
ORDERING INFORMATION	Available from The National Audiovisual Center.
PRICE	Free.

A LIST of AUDIOVISUAL MATERIALS PRODUCED by the UNITED STATES GOVERNMENT for FIRE/LAW ENFORCEMENT

National Audiovisual Center, National Archives and Records Service. U.S. General Services Administration. 1980. 21 p.

MEDIA	16mm films, filmstrips, videocassettes, slide sets, audiotapes, multimedia kits.
SUMMARY	This directory contains 190 audiovisuals produced by the U.S. Government for fire or law enforcement. Specific areas covered are: disaster preparedness, emergency medical service, fire prevention, law enforcement, wildfire, and new and noteworthy items. Most entries are current, with a few dating back as far as 1959.
ENTRIES	Title, running time or number of frames, format, sound or silent, color or b/w, year of release, producer, title number, sale price, annotation, TV clearance, language (if other than English).
SPECIAL FEATURES	Gives information on other catalogs published by the National Audiovisual Center, ordering information, information on public services by the Center. Title index is also included.
ORDERING INFORMATION	Available from The National Audiovisual Center.
PRICE	Free.

A LIST of AUDIOVISUAL MATERIALS PRODUCED by the UNITED STATES GOVERNMENT for FLIGHT and METEOROLOGY

National Audiovisual Center, National Archives and Records Service. U.S. General Services Administration. August 15, 1980. 15 p.

MEDIA	16mm films, filmstrips, videocassettes, audiotapes.
SUMMARY	This directory contains approximately 150 audiovisuals produced by the U.S. Government for flight and meteorology. Some specific subjects covered are: aero-medical problems, air accidents, care and safety precautions to be used in handling toxic chemicals used in aerial applications, disorientation, effects of altitude on humans, effects of drinking and alcoholism on the job, hurricane preparedness, hypoxia, medical facts in flying, including the physical, psychological, and physiological limitations, safety, vision requirements, and weather conditions affecting the aircraft and personnel. Film entries which have been produced beginning in 1940 to the pre-space era and considered of historical value are also included.
ENTRIES	Title, format, running time or number of frames, year of release, agency's number, sound or silent, sale price, annotation, TV clearance, language, audience level, series.
SPECIAL FEATURES	Gives information on other catalogs published by the National Audiovisual Center, ordering information, and information on public services by the Center. Title index is also included.
ORDERING INFORMATION	Available from The National Audiovisual Center.
PRICE	Free.

A LIST of AUDIOVISUAL MATERIALS PRODUCED by the UNITED STATES GOVERNMENT for FOREIGN LANGUAGE INSTRUCTION

National Audiovisual Center, National Archives and Records Service. U.S. General Services Administration. February 15, 1980. 7 p.

MEDIA	Audiotapes with print text.
SUMMARY	This directory contains 1,570 audiotapes produced by the U.S. Government for foreign language instruction. These materials can be used for teaching foreign health professionals or persons who do government and volunteer work in other countries, both during war and for humanitarian purposes. Teaching materials in forty different languages have been produced and listed. Specific languages included are: Amharic, Arabic, Baluchi, Bulgarian, Cambodian, Cantonese, Chinyanja, Finnish, French, Fula, German, Greek, Hausa, Hebrew, Hungarian, Igbo, Italian, Japanese, Kirundi, Kituba, Korean, Lao, Lingala, Luganda, Mandarin, More, Portuguese, Serbo-Croatian, Shona, Sinhalese, Spanish, Standard Chinese, Swahili, Swedish, Thai, Turkish, Twi, Urdu, Vietnamese, and Yoruba.
ENTRIES	Language, course title, unit(s), number of tapes, track(s), ID number for tapes, accompanying print material (text), sale price per unit, availability information. (n.d.)
SPECIAL FEATURES	Includes glossary section, information on other catalogs published by the National Audiovisual Center, information on additional services from the Center, ordering information.
ORDERING INFORMATION	Available from The National Audiovisual Center.
PRICE	Free.

A LIST of AUDIOVISUAL MATERIALS PRODUCED by the UNITED STATES GOVERNMENT for INDUSTRIAL SAFETY

National Audiovisual Center, National Archives and Records Service. U.S. General Services Administration. April 15, 1980. 18 p.

MEDIA	16mm films, filmstrips, videocassettes, slide sets, audiotapes, multimedia kits.
SUMMARY	This directory contains 138 audiovisuals produced by the U.S. Government for industrial safety. Specific areas of safety coverage include: agriculture, first aid, industry, laboratory, materials handling, and mining. In the Miscellaneous Section, audiovisuals on fire and fire safety, noise pollution, safety regulations, hazards of LNG spills in marine transportation, and orientation programs in occupational safety and health for federal employees are also included. Most of the materials are current but items considered of historical value are also contained in the directory.
ENTRIES	Title, running time or number of frames, format, sound or silent, color or b/w, year of release, producer, title number, sale price, annotation, TV clearance, language (if other than English).
SPECIAL FEATURES	Gives information on other catalogs published by the National Audiovisual Center, title index, ordering information, and information on public services by the Center.
ORDERING INFORMATION	Available from The National Audiovisual Center.
PRICE	Free.

A LIST of AUDIOVISUAL MATERIALS PRODUCED by the UNITED STATES GOVERNMENT for NURSING

National Audiovisual Center, National Archives and Records Service. U.S. General Services Administration. August 15, 1980. 15 p.

MEDIA	16mm films, filmstrips, videocassettes, slide sets, audiotapes, multimedia kits.
SUMMARY	This directory contains 137 audiovisuals produced by the U.S. Government for nursing. Specific subjects included are: basic patient care, handicapped patients, medical procedures, mental illness, and the nursing profession.
ENTRIES	Title, running time or number of frames, format, sound or silent, color or b/w, year of release, TV clearance, language (if other than English).
SPECIAL FEATURES	Gives information on other catalogs published by the National Audiovisual Center, ordering information, information on public services by the Center. Title index is also included.
ORDERING INFORMATION	Available from The National Audiovisual Center.
PRICE	Free.

A LIST of AUDIOVISUAL MATERIALS PRODUCED by the UNITED STATES GOVERNMENT for SOCIAL ISSUES

National Audiovisual Center, National Archives and Records Service. U.S. General Services Administration. June 1, 1980. 20 p.

MEDIA	16mm films, filmstrips, videocassettes, slide sets, audiotapes, multimedia kits.
SUMMARY	This directory contains 175 audiovisuals produced by the U.S. Government for social issues. Specific areas of coverage include: aging, child abuse, death and bereavement, human relations, mental health and psychology, minorities, parenting, social work, and women. All of the entries are current and should be of particular value to social workers.
ENTRIES	Title, running time or number of frames, format, sound or silent, color or b/w, year of release, producer, title number, sale price, annotation, TV clearance, language (if other than English).
SPECIAL FEATURES	Gives information on other catalogs published by the National Audiovisual Center, ordering information, information on public services by the Center. Title index is also included.
ORDERING INFORMATION	Available from The National Audiovisual Center.
PRICE	Free.

A LIST of AUDIOVISUAL MATERIALS PRODUCED by the UNITED STATES GOVERNMENT for SPECIAL EDUCATION

National Audiovisual Center, National Archives and Records Service. U.S. General Services Administration. June 16, 1980. 25 p.

MEDIA	16mm films, filmstrips, videocassettes, slide sets, audiotapes, multimedia kits.
SUMMARY	This directory contains 165 audiovisuals produced by the U.S. Government for special education. Specific areas covered are: captioned films, films for the emotionally disturbed, general films with broad content, the handicapped adult, the hearing impaired, human development, manual communication, mental retardation, parent education, the physically handicapped, and speech and language development. All entries are current, with production dates beginning in 1970 to the present.
ENTRIES	Time, running time or number of frames, format, sound or silent, color or b/w, year of release, producer, title number, sale price, annotation, TV clearance, language (if other than English).
SPECIAL FEATURES	Includes information on additional services available from the National Audiovisual Center, ordering information, borrowing policies, and a section on captioned films for the deaf. Title index is also included.
ORDERING INFORMATION	Available from The National Audiovisual Center.
PRICE	Free.

A LIST of AUDIOVISUAL MATERIALS PRODUCED by the UNITED STATES GOVERNMENT in HISTORY

National Audiovisual Center, National Archives and Records Service. U.S. General Services Administration. [1980]. 20 p.

MEDIA	16mm films, filmstrips, videocasettes, slide sets, audiotapes, multimedia kits.
SUMMARY	This directory contains 310 audiovisuals produced by the U.S. Government in history. Both new items and footage reflecting past wars such as World Wars I and II, the Korean and the Vietnam wars are included. Many film entries have won numerous awards, including Academy Awards. Among subject areas covered are: between war activities, crimes against humanity, the discovery of plutonium in the Fermi laboratory, effects of dropping the hydrogen bomb on humans and environment, evacuation, first aid during war, hospitals overseas during wars, medical programs, nursing in the army, rescue procedures, war disasters, and war hazards.
ENTRIES	Title, running time or number of frames, format, sound or silent, color or b/w, year of release, producer, title number, sale price, annotation, TV clearance, language (if other than English), special notes to users, series, awards.
SPECIAL FEATURES	This directory includes monumental, documentary films such as "The Plow that Broke the Plains" (1936), "The River" (1939) produced by the Department of Agriculture, "Seeds of Destiny" (1947) produced by the War Department, and other documentary films which became a landmark in motion picture-making.
ORDERING INFORMATION	Available from The National Audiovisual Center.
PRICE	Free.

A LIST of AUDIOVISUAL MATERIALS PRODUCED by the UNITED STATES GOVERNMENT—SPANISH LANGUAGE SOUNDTRACKS

National Audiovisual Center, National Archives and Records Service. U.S. General Services Administration. 1980. 13 p.

MEDIA	16mm films, filmstrips, videocassettes, slide sets, audiotapes, multimedia kits.
SUMMARY	This directory includes 130 audiovisual materials produced by the U.S. Government with Spanish language soundtracks. Area coverage feature: business and management, drugs and alcohol, cardiopulmonary resuscitation (CPR), education and training, emergencies, nutrition, pest control, psychology and social problems, vocational and technical materials. Some entries date back to 1944, but most are current.
ENTRIES	Title, running time or number of frames, format, sound or silent, color or b/w, year of release, producer, title number, sale price, annotation, TV clearance, language (if other than English).
SPECIAL FEATURES	Gives information on other catalogs published by the National Audiovisual Center, ordering information, information on public services by the Center. Title index is also included.
ORDERING INFORMATION	Available from The National Audiovisual Center.
PRICE	Free.

LIST of EDUCATIONAL AIDS

U.S. Armed Forces Institute of Pathology. June 1981. Announcements. Veterinary Pathology List. 1981. 24 p.

MEDIA	16mm films, lantern slide sets, microscopic slides.
SUMMARY	This union list of approximately 2,500 educational materials produced by the military and federal agencies for their use, are also made available to civilian professionals, medical residents, and physicians in all specialties. Subject areas included are: aerospace animal studies, asbestos-related diseases, basic sciences, cardiovascular, dental and oral diagnostic problems, drug interaction, embryology, endocrine, forensic medicine, gastro-intestinal, general pathology, genitourinary, hematologic, hepatic, histochemistry, historical sciences of the Army, infectious diseases, laboratory training, lasers, microscope (use), neuropathology, nurse corps, nutrition, ophthalmic, orthopedic, otorhinolaryngology, pediatrics, pulmonary, skin soft tissue, surgery and surgical pathology, tissue reactions to drugs, veterinary. Pictorial atlas of tumor pathology is also included. This edition includes a section entitled VETERINARY PATHOLOGY LOAN STUDY SETS in the AFIP Loan Service, which includes over 100 slide sets available for loan. Some of the entries date back to 1940.
ENTRIES	Letter of identification (format), accession number, title, running time or number of frames, sound or silent, color or b/w, year of release, producer.
SPECIAL FEATURES	Includes instructions to the users, special instructions to foreign requestors included in the supplement, subject index and order forms. Atlas of tumor pathology with prices is also included.
ORDERING INFORMATION	Available from the Superintendent of Documents, U.S. Government Printing Office: 1974 0-557-94.
PRICE	$2.05.

LISTING of EDUCATIONAL MATERIALS for USE by SCHOOLS

Office of Communications, Division of Consumer Education and Awareness. U.S. Consumer Product Safety Commission. 1978. 14 p.

MEDIA	16mm films, slide sets.
SUMMARY	Includes 15 programs accompanied by manuals developed by the U.S. Consumer Product Safety Commission especially for use by educators in teaching safety to youngsters. Topics included are: baby sitters safety, bicycle safety, burns/prevention, child/nursery furniture safety, flammable products safety, kitchen safety, lawn mower safety, outdoor playground equipment safety, poison prevention, and toy safety. These programs are available on a free loan basis from 27 libraries of Modern Talking Pictures, Inc. Some of the audiovisuals are also available from the Commission's 13 area offices listed in this catalog.
ENTRIES	Title, grade level, parts of the package, format, color or b/w, running time or number of frames, availability information.
SPECIAL FEATURES	Includes a list of Consumer Product Safety Commission area offices and a list of Modern Talking Pictures Libraries, year of release (when available).
ORDERING INFORMATION	Available from the Superintendent of Documents, U.S. Government Printing Office: 1978-720-332/3918 or the U.S. Consumer Product Safety Commission.
PRICE	Free.

MEDIA RESOURCES CATALOG

Media Services Center, Bureau of Prisons. U.S. Department of Justice. August, 1977. 58 p.

(This publication was printed by Federal Prison Industries, Inc., Printing Plant, Federal Correctional Institution, Lompoc, California.)

MEDIA	16mm films, videocassettes, slide sets.
SUMMARY	This catalog contains approximately 60 current programs produced by both U.S. Government and independent producers in the United States and abroad. Among the entries designed for those in the field of corrections and personnel management, broad health sciences, subject categories are also included: behavioral sciences, counseling, FDA report on drug abuse, handicapped, homosexuality, law enforcement, mental health, physical education, prison life, rape, rehabilitation, research.
ENTRIES	Title, format, color or b/w, running time or number of frames, year of release, annotation, producer, availability.
SPECIAL FEATURES	Includes order form and title index.
ORDERING INFORMATION	Available from the U.S. Bureau of Prisons. Publication FPI-LOM 9-30-77.
PRICE	Free.

MEDICAL CATALOG of SELECTED AUDIOVISUAL MATERIALS PRODUCED by the UNITED STATES GOVERNMENT*

National Audiovisual Center, National Archives and Records Service. U.S. General Services Administration. 1980. 187 p.

MEDIA	16mm films, filmstrips, videocassettes, slide sets, audiotapes, multimedia kits.
SUMMARY	Lists more than 2,000 medical and allied health audiovisuals materials representing one of the major subject concentrations in the Center's collection of more than 13,000 federally produced audiovisuals. Available for purchase, rent, and loan from the National Audiovisual Center. Major subject areas covered are: agriculture, atomic energy, aviation, biology, business and economics, chemistry, civics and government, computer science, dentistry, drug abuse, education, electronics, engineering, environmental health, fine arts, forestry, health, health related occupations, library science, medicine, military and naval science, nursing, nutrition, physical fitness, plastic and reconstructive surgery, pollution, rehabilitation, safety, sex education, smoking, sociology, space programs, surgery, urbanization, and wounds and injuries. Many entries date back to 1940.
ENTRIES	Title, running time or number of frames, format, sound or silent, b/w, producer, year of release, number assigned by the producing agency, availability, annotation, series notes, additional notes on use or production.
SPECIAL FEATURES	Gives information on audiovisual services, productions, and publications of the National Audiovisual Center and individual Federal agencies. Includes Subject Section, Sponsor/Producer codes, purchase, rental, and loan policies, and price lists. In various pages describes the collection of materials produced and distributed by the U.S. Government. An outline of subject headings is also included.
ORDERING INFORMATION	Available from the Superintendent of Documents, U.S. Government Printing Office: Stock number 022-002-00066-0.
PRICE	$6.00.

MEDICAL FILM CATALOG

Naval Health Sciences Education and Training Command and National Naval Medical Center, Audiovisual Resource Section. U.S. Navy. 1974. [127] p.

MEDIA	16mm films, videocassettes.
SUMMARY	This catalog includes approximately 800 audiovisual materials produced for the U.S. Navy by both U.S. Government agencies and independent producers, covering all aspects of medicine and allied health. These materials are classified under the following broad subjects: aerospace medicine, anatomy, anesthesiology, dermatology, drugs and drug abuse, ear, nose, throat, ecology, energy, first aid, global medicine, history of medicine, internal medicine, laboratory techniques, management and hospital administration, military medicine, naval medical careers, neurology and neurosurgery, nuclear/biological/chemical (NBC) operations, nuclear medicine, obstetrics and gynecology, ophthalmology, orthopedics, pathology, patient care, pediatrics, physical medicine and rehabilitation, physiology, plastic surgery, polar medicine, preventive medicine, psychiatry, radiation, radiology, safety, sanitation, submarine and diving medicine, surgery (general), tropical medicine, veterinary medicine. Most of the materials are current but some date back to 1940.
ENTRIES	Title, series, producer, film number, format, color or b/w, sound or silent, running time, year of release, annotation, viewing restrictions.
SPECIAL FEATURES	Includes ordering information and forms, title, subject, and topical indexes.
ORDERING INFORMATION	Available from the Audiovisual Resources Section, Naval Health Sciences Education and Training Command, National Naval Medical Center. U.S. Navy.
PRICE	Free.

MENTAL RETARDATION FILM LIST

Social Rehabilitation Service. U.S. Department of Health, Education, and Welfare. [1968]. 60 p.

(This publication was prepared for the Division of Mental Retardation, Social and Rehabilitation Service, by the National Medical Audiovisual Center, National Library of Medicine, Public Health Service.)

MEDIA	16mm and 36mm films, filmstrips, slide sets, audiotapes, recordings.
SUMMARY	Contains annotated entries for 150 selected audiovisuals for use in mental retardation education programs. Entries are divided into two groups: Nonprofessional films intended for use by the general public and concerning the nature of mental retardation, its causes, general treatment, and prevention; and Professional films dealing with more specific aspects of diagnosis, clinical treatment, rehabilitation, and control. Includes materials produced and distributed by U.S., foreign governments, and private agencies. Some films date back to 1950.
ENTRIES	Title, producer/distributor, country of origin, year of release, edition, running time, sound or silent, color or b/w, format, accompanying materials, language, series, annotation, sale source, distributor.
SPECIAL FEATURES	Includes borrowing information, list of distributors, and title index.
ORDERING INFORMATION	Available from the National Medical Audiovisual Center.
PRICE	Free.

NASA FILM LIST

U.S. National Aeronautics and Space Administration. January 1976. 28 p.

MEDIA	16mm films, filmstrips, audiotapes.
SUMMARY	This catalog includes 80 audiovisuals produced by the National Aeronautics and Space Administration for public use, which cover the following topics: advanced emergency systems, agricultural studies, atmospheric studies, collection of soil from the moon, computer program (NASTRAN) for solving structural engineering design problems in industry, history of space flight, international cooperation in the development of spacelab, life on other planets, life-or-death problems in aerospace, mass radiation, NASA's efforts in extending the benefits of its research in medicine, natural and man-made disasters, paramedics, personal hygiene in waste disposal, pollution, presentations of works of prominent anthropologists, safety/aerospace, studies of the solar system, telecare, teamwork in overcoming disasters in spacecraft. Because of the continuing research and discovery in many areas of space and aeronautics programs, the information contained in some of NASA films might seem dated, but they are included because of their historical interest. The catalog is divided in the following sections: NASA films of general interest, general films, rediscovery series, educational and special interest films for non-technical audience, adventure in research, NASA filmstrips, NASA audiotapes, space in the 70's series. All materials are available for public viewing.
ENTRIES	Title, ordering number, year of release, color or b/w, running time or number of frames, annotation, awards.
SPECIAL FEATURES	Includes a list of NASA Regional Film Libraries, information on loan or purchase, prices, and alphabetical index within each section.
ORDERING INFORMATION	Available from the Superintendent of Documents, U.S. Government Printing Office: 1076-0-2-1-182.
PRICE	Free.

NATIONAL LIBRARY of MEDICINE AUDIOVISUALS CATALOG*

National Library of Medicine, National Institutes of Health, Public Health Service. U.S. Department of Health, Education, and Welfare. 1977-. (Quarterly, January-March, April-June, July-September, and Annual Cumulation January-December.)

MEDIA | 16mm films, videocassettes.

SUMMARY | This catalog is a cumulation of audiovisual materials cataloged by the National Library of Medicine during the year. These audiovisuals are produced by both Government agencies and independent producers and are available from sources cited in each entry. The catalog is divided into two general categories: (1) Includes materials developed for use in the health-science education. All these materials have been reviewed by subject specialists, under the auspices of the Association of Medical Colleges. All entries in this section include abstracts (annotations). (2) These lecture-type materials represent the recording of educational events—lectures, congresses, symposia, grand rounds, etc. These materials are not reviewed by subject specialists, but do contain full bibliographic and ordering information with no abstracts. All materials are classifed under subject headings from *Medical Education Headings (MeSH)*, NLM's controlled vocabulary used in the preparation of *Index Medicus* as well as for subject cataloging in the NLM *Current Catalog*. Earlier materials appeared in the NLM AVLINE, 1975-1976 issues. AVLINE is available for search and retrieval at over 1,000 institutions which belong to NLM's online network. Broad subject categories included are: accidents and their prevention, alcohol and alcoholism, anatomy, anesthesiology, animal(s), behavioral sciences, biology, cancer/neoplasms, cardiovascular system, chemistry, child abuse, communicable diseases, cytology and tissue culture, death, dentistry, dermatology, digestive system, disasters, drugs and drug abuse, education (medical), electronics (medical), embryology, endocrine system, environment (life style/occupational), epidemiology, first aid, genetics, geriatrics (aging), growth (human and primates), gynecology, hemic and lymphatic systems, heredity, history of medicine, human development, hypertension, industrial medicine, health (occupational), mental retardation, microbiology, military medicine, musculoskeletal system, nervous system, nursing and patient care, obstetrics, occupational therapy, ophthalmology, otorhinolaryngology, pediatrics, pharmacology and pharmacognosy, physical fitness, physical medicine, preventive medicine, physical therapy, psychiatry and psychology, respiratory system, sex education, smoking, social sciences, surgery, technology (industrial, agriculture, food), thanatology, toxicology, urogenital system, veterinary medicine, world health, wounds and injuries, zoology. Most of the programs are current but some earlier productions are also included.

ENTRIES	In section one: title, producer, year of release, sound or silent, color or b/w, format, audience level, specialty, accompanying print material, credits, annotation, subject headings, series, availability information, item number. Section two (name/title section): main heading, subheading (format), title, format, corporate body or person, year of release, running time, sound or silent, size (width), credits, audience, subject(s), review (reviewer, date), NLM call number, source (procurement), unique citation ID number.
SPECIAL FEATURES	Includes: (a) monographs subject section; (b) monographs name and title section; (c) serials subject section; (d) serials name and title section; (e) procurement section.
ORDERING INFORMATION	Available from the Superintendent of Documents, U.S. Government Printing Office on Subscription.
PRICE	Domestic—$24.00; Foreign—$30.00. 1977 annual cumulation. Issues as part of the NLM Audiovisuals Catalog (quarterly), is also available separately. Price: $11.00 ($13.75 foreign). (NOTE: When ordering include words "4th quarter, 1979") HE 20: 3609/4:979/4; 1978 $10.00 ($13.75 foreign). S/N 017-052-72074-1. 1980 annual cumulation $11.00 ($13.75 foreign). S/N 017-052-72090-2. 1981 Subscription (3 quarterlies, plus annual cumulation), $24.00 ($30.00). Send subscriptions to the (AV), National Library of Medicine, Bethesda, Maryland 20209.

NATIONAL LIBRARY of MEDICINE AVLINE CATALOG, 1975-1976*

National Library of Medicine, National Institutes of Health, Public Health Service. U.S. Department of Health, Education, and Welfare, 1977. 339. (Updates, covering items catalog in 1977 or later, appear quarterly in the NLM CURRENT CATALOG.)

MEDIA	16mm, 35mm films, filmstrips, audiocassettes, slide sets, audiotapes, multimedia kits, recordings.
SUMMARY	Presents bibliography and review data of approximately 2,400 audiovisual packages in the health sciences at the college level and for the continuing educational practitioners, as cataloged by NLM from November 1975 through December 1976 for its AVLINE (Audiovisuals On-Line) database. The materials are designed to assist the fulfillment of national teaching and learning objectives. Audiovisuals are produced by U.S. Government agencies, medical schools, colleges and universities, professional associations, and independent producers. All entries have been professionally reviewed for technical quality, currency, educational design, and accuracy under the auspices of the Association of American Medical Colleges and the American Association of Dental Schools. Broad subjects included are: accidents and accident prevention, administration (hospital, medical), alcohol and alcoholism, anatomy, anesthesiology, arthritis, biology, body as a whole, cancer/neoplasms, cardiovascular system, chemistry, child abuse, communicable diseases, cytology, and tissue culture, dentistry, dermatology, digestive system, disasters, drugs and drug abuse, education (medical), embryology, endocrine system, environment (social) and environmental health, evolution (human and non-human primates), eye, first aid, genetics, geriatrics, hemic and lymphatic systems, heredity, history of medicine, human development (evolution), hypertension, industrial medicine (occupational), microbiology, military medicine, musculoskeletal system, nursing and patient care. otorhinolaryngology, pediatrics, pharmacology and pharmacognosy, physical fitness, physiology, psychiatry and psychology, preventive medicine, public health, radiology, rehabilitation, respiratory system, sex education, smoking (tobacco), social sciences, surgery, technology (industrial, agricultural, food), thanatology, toxicology, urogenital system, veterinary medicine, world health, zoology. AVLINE is available for search and retrieval at over 1,000 institutions in the United States which belong to NLM's online network. Materials are listed under terms selected from the National Library of Medicine's Medical Subject Headings (MeSH). For titles in fields peripheral to medicine, Library of Congress classification schedules are used.

ENTRIES	Heading, related subject heading(s), subject heading with format, title, medium (format), body or person responsible for the work, sale or loan source, number of reels, running time or number of frames, sound or silent, series, audience, review data, credits, NLM call number, rental and purchase prices, information for loan, procurement source(s), unique citation ID number.
SPECIAL FEATURES	Includes notes for catalogers and a list of distributors (procurement section).
ORDERING INFORMATION	Available from the National Technical Information Service (NTIS), U.S. Department of Commerce. DHEW Publication No. (NIH) 77-1295.
PRICE	$5.00. ($6.50 foreign.)

NATIONAL MEDICAL AUDIOVISUAL CENTER CATALOG: FILMS for the HEALTH SCIENCES*

National Medical Audiovisual Center, National Library of Medicine, National Institutes of Health, Public Health Service. U.S. Department of Health, Education, and Welfare. 1981. Plus announcements.

MEDIA   16mm films (also available in ¾" videocassette format and videotape).

SUMMARY   This catalog contains more than 700 16mm motion pictures included in the Library of Medicine's computerized data base, AVLINE (Audio-visuals-on-Line). The national Medical Audiovisual Center (NMAC), a component of the National Library of Medicine (NLM), acquires and distributes evaluated audiovisual material and also conducts a series of programs in media development, consultation, training, and educational research. All these programs are aimed at increasing the effectiveness of medical education by developing innovative instructional material and promoting the sharing of materials among the national and international health sciences educational communities. All films are also available on a free-loan basis to foreign countries included in the U.S. Agency for International Development/National Library of Medicine Agreement.[1] Requesters in non-AID foreign countries are required to pay a fee of $10.00. All materials have been professionally reviewed for technical quality, currency, educational design, and accuracy under the auspices of the Association of American Medical Colleges and the American Association of Dental Schools. The catalog is divided into two sections: The Subject Section with entries listed under terms selected from the NLM's Medical Subject Headings (MeSH), and Name/Title Section with entries listed alphabetically by the first significant word and containing the full citation. This comprehensive catalog includes all productions of historical value dating back to 1929. Broad subject categories included are: accidents, alcohol and alcoholism, anatomy, anesthesiology, animal(s), arthritis, behavioral sciences, biology, cancer/neoplasms, cardiovascular system, chemistry, child abuse, communicable diseases, cytology and tissue culture, death, dentistry, dermatology, digestive system, drugs and drug abuse, education (medical), electronics (medical), embryology, endocrine system, environment (life style and occupational), epidemiology,

---

[1]The Agency for International Development (AID) carries out assistance programs designed to help people of developing countries develop their human and economic resources, increase productive capabilities, and improve the quality of human life as well as to promote the economics of political stability in friendly countries." *The United States Government Manual* 1981/1981. Office of the Registar, National Archives and Records Service. U.S. General Services Administration, 1981. p. 633. [For the Agency of International Development statement or organization see *Federal Register* of Aug. 14, 1980, 45 FR 54149-5444].

first aid, genetics, geriatrics, growth (human and primates), gynecology, hemic and lymphatic systems, heredity, history of medicine, human development, hypertension, industrial medicine (occupational), microbiology, military medicine, musculoskeletal system, nervous system, nursing and patient care, obstetrics, occupational therapy, ophthalmology, otorhinolaryngcology, pediatrics, pharmacology and pharmacognosy, physical fitness, physical medicine, preventive medicine, psychiatry and psychology, public health, pulmonary medicine, radiology, rehabilitation, respiratory system, sex education, social sciences, surgery, technology (industrial, agricultural, food), thanatology, toxicology, urogenital system, world health, wounds and injuries, zoology.

ENTRIES Title, producer, year of release, running time, sound or silent, color or b/w, format, audience level, specialty(s), accompanying print material, credits, annotation, subject headings, series, availability information, item number.

SPECIAL FEATURES Includes information to eligible users, ordering instructions, note to catalogers and order forms. Subject index is also included.

ORDERING INFORMATION Available from the Superintendent of Documents, U.S. Government Printing Office: S/N 017-052-00221-0.

PRICE Domestic—$7.00; Foreign—plus $1.75.

NEUROLOGICAL and SENSORY DISEASE FILM GUIDE, 1966

Neurological and Sensory Disease Service Program, Division of Chronic Diseases, Public Health Service. U.S. Department of Health, Education, and Welfare. 1966. 220 p.

MEDIA	16mm films, filmstrips, slide sets.
SUMMARY	This catalog lists 1,348 audiovisuals selected primarily to help medical and allied health professional teaching institutions, hospitals, and other users to find educational material related to the field of medicine. Among the 29 neurological diseases included are: cerebral palsy, epilepsy, mental retardation, and speech disorders. Sensory diseases of the ear, eye, larynx, nose, and speech with their diagnosis and treatment are also included.
ENTRIES	Title, producer, country of origin, year of release, running time or number of frames, sound or silent, color or b/w, language (if other than English), credits, availability information, sale or purchase price, annotation, reviews.
SPECIAL FEATURES	Includes distributor list, list of categories, subject listing, title listing, and order form.
ORDERING INFORMATION	Available from the National Technical Information Service (NTIS), PHS Publication No. 1033.
PRICE	$3.50.

NIOSH—FILMS and FILMSTRIPS on OCCUPATIONAL SAFETY and HEALTH

National Institute of Occupational Safety and Health, Center for Disease Control, Public Health Service. U.S. Department of Health, Education, and Welfare. 1975. [52] p. Plus supplements and announcements.

MEDIA	16mm films, filmstrips, slide sets.
SUMMARY	This catalog includes approximately 150 audiovisual programs covering all aspects of occupational safety and health, produced by the U.S. Government agencies, independent producers, and organizations. Subjects include: chemicals, construction and plant safety, electricity, equipment, eyes and vision, falls/slips/backs, fire and explosion, general safety, hospitals, nursing, industrial hygiene, industrial medicine, laboratory safety, lead, mercury, mining, noise, pesticides, power tools, protective devices, radiation, skin, supervision, welding. Some of these materials, which are available to the public from NIOSH, date back to 1940.
ENTRIES	Title, format, sound or silent, color or b/w, running time or number of frames, year of release (when available), annotation, distributor other than NIOSH.
SPECIAL FEATURES	Includes ordering information for both NIOSH and independent distributors, and a list of organizations providing rental or sale films and filmstrips dealing with occupational safety and health.
ORDERING INFORMATION	Available from the Superintendent of Documents, U.S. Government Printing Office: 1975-657-601/5540 Region No. 5-11/HEW Publication No. (NIOSH) 75-128.
PRICE	Single copy available from NIOSH.

1970 FILM REFERENCE GUIDE for MEDICINE and ALLIED HEALTH SCIENCES

National Medical Audiovisual Center, National Library of Medicine, National Institutes of Health, Public Health Service. U.S. Department of Health, Education, and Welfare. 1970. [311] p.

MEDIA	8mm, 16mm, 35mm films, filmstrips, slide sets, audiotapes, recordings.
SUMMARY	This guide was sponsored and published by the Federal Advisory Council on Medical Training Aids (FACMTA) to provide a basic catalog of selected audiovisuals used in biomedical education primarily by member agencies. Includes approximately 2,000 entries produced by both U.S. Government agencies and independent producers for distribution throughout the world. Major subject areas covered are: accidents and accident prevention, alcohol and drug addiction, agriculture, aviation medicine, biology, cancer, cardiovascular system, chemistry, child care and maternal welfare, cosmetic surgery, civil defense and disaster, digestive system, ear, environmental sciences, first aid, food, forensic medicine, gerontology, international health, nursing, nutrition, hospital and medical facilities, pharmacology and toxicology, psychiatry and psychology, radiology, sanitary engineering, sex education, surgery, urogenital system, veterinary medicine, zoology. Includes items which have been produced since 1940 but are medically sound and carry historical value.
ENTRIES	Title, producer/sponsor, country of origin, year of release, releasing agent, series title (if any), running time or number of frames, color or b/w, sound or silent, format, distributor(s), credits, availability information, annotation.
SPECIAL FEATURES	Includes instructions for borrowing audiovisuals, distributor list, and subject index.
ORDERING INFORMATION	Available from the National Technical Information Service (NTIS), PHS No. 476, Revised 1970.
PRICE	$3.50.

1969 FILM REFERENCE GUIDE for MEDICINE and ALLIED SCIENCES

National Medical Audiovisual Center, National Library of Medicine, National Institutes of Health, Public Health Service. U.S. Department of Health, Education, and Welfare. 1968. 386 p. 1969 Supplement, 74 p.

MEDIA	8mm, 16mm, 35mm films, filmstrips, audiotapes, recordings.
SUMMARY	This guide was sponsored and published by the Federal Advisory Council on Medical Training Aids (FACTMA). Includes approximately 5,000 medical audiovisual programs, selected from 9,000 motion pictures, 8,000 filmstrips, and 1,300 audiotapes of the U.S. Public Health Service Audiovisual Center's collection produced by both U.S. Government agencies and independent producers from all over the world. Major subject areas covered are: accidents and accident prevention, addiction, agriculture, biology, cancer, cardiovascular system, chemistry, child care and maternal welfare, civil defense, dentistry, digestive system, ear, environmental sciences, first aid, international health, microbiology, nursing, nutrition, occupational health, pharmacology and toxicology, psychiatry, psychology, radiology, surgery, veterinary medicine. Some entries date back to 1940 but carry historical value.
ENTRIES	Title, producer/sponsor, country of origin, year of release, releasing agent, series title (if any), running time or number of frames, color or b/w, sound or silent, format, distributor(s), credits, annotation.
SPECIAL FEATURES	Includes instructions for borrowing audiovisuals, distributor list, corrigenda, and subject index.
ORDERING INFORMATION	Available from the National Technical Information Service (NTIS), NIH Publication 451.
PRICE	1968, $3.50; 1969, $1.70 (Supplement).

1967 PUBLIC HEALTH SERVICE FILM CATALOG

National Medical Audiovisual Center, National Library of Medicine, Public Health Service. U.S. Department of Health, Education, and Welfare. 1967. 103 p.

MEDIA	16mm, 35mm films, filmstrips, audiotapes.
SUMMARY	Includes approximately 1,000 entries selected for use in the medical programs. Major subjects covered are: accident and accident prevention, addiction, agriculture, allergy, body as a whole, biology, cancer, cardiovascular system, chemistry, child care and maternal welfare, civil defense, dentistry, digestive system, environmental sciences, ear, first aid, food, hospital and medical facilities, international health, microbiology, nursing, nutrition, occupational health, pharmacology and toxicology, plastic surgery, psychiatry and psychology, rehabilitation, surgery, radiology, sanitary engineering, veterinary medicine, water supply and pollution control.
ENTRIES	Title, order number, producer/sponsor, year of release, revised, running time or number of frames, sound or silent, color or b/w, format, kinescope, accompanying print material, language (if other than English), annotation, credits.
SPECIAL FEATURES	Includes subject and title indexes.
ORDERING INFORMATION	Available from the National Technical Information Service (NTIS), PHS Publication No. 776.
PRICE	$3.50.

NOAA MOTION PICTURE FILMS

National Oceanic and Atmospheric Administration. U.S. Department of Commerce. 1978. 15 p. Plus announcements.

MEDIA	16mm films.
SUMMARY	This pamphlet includes 53 films produced and distributed free of charge by the National Oceanic and Atmospheric Administration. Subject areas covered by these films are: aerospace, environmental sciences, fish cookery, fishery conservation, global weather experiments (environmental satellites), history of satellites, marine biology, meteorological and oceanographic activities, natural disasters, oceanic general sciences, research programs such as Global Atmospheric Research (GARP), and Atlantic Tropical Experiment (GATE).
ENTRIES	Title/General Topic, running time, color, annotation, and pictorial sketch representing topic.
SPECIAL INFORMATION	Includes borrowing information, title index, and pictures.
ORDERING INFORMATION	Available from the National Oceanic and Atmospheric Administration.
PRICE	Free.

PUBLICATIONS, RADIO, FILMS, SLIDES, FACT SHEETS, T.V.

Consumer Product Safety Commission. U.S. Consumer Product Safety Commission. 1976. 16 p.

MEDIA	16mm films, filmstrips, slide sets, fact sheets.
SUMMARY	Includes 25 entries concerning the laws administered by the Consumer Product Safety Commission in all aspects of product safety. Specific subject areas covered are: bicycles, cribs, flammable fabrics, household products, outdoor power equipment, packaging and toys safety, poison prevention, and product safety education. Programs on general information for the public, the Hazardous Substances Act, the National Injury Surveillance System (NISS), and radio spots providing guidance on selection, use and maintenance of infant nursery equipment are also included. These audiovisuals are available from designated film libraries around the country. Print materials are available from the U.S. Consumer Product Safety Commission. Some materials are also available in Spanish.
ENTRIES	Title, running time or number of frames, color or b/w, sound or silent, annotation, audience level, sale price, distributor.
SPECIAL FEATURES	Includes information about the Commission's activities, list of free publications and their sources, list of distributing film libraries. A list of Consumer Product Safety Commission Offices around the country is also included.
ORDERING INFORMATION	Available from the Consumer Product Safety Commission or from the U.S. Government Printing Office: 1976. CPSC Publication 77-620-9.
PRICE	Free.

QUARTERLY UPDATE: A COMPREHENSIVE LISTING of NEW AUDIOVISUAL MATERIALS and SERVICES OFFERED by the NATIONAL AUDIOVISUAL CENTER*

National Audiovisual Center, National Archives and Records Service. U.S. General Services Administration. October, 1980.

(Indefinitely discontinued after two issues of June and October, 1980.)

MEDIA	16mm films, filmstrips, videocassettes, slides and slide sets, audiotapes, multimedia kits.
SUMMARY	The Quarterly Update includes all recent additions of productions in all subject areas of the National Audiovisual Center's collection. Titles are listed under general subjects and include a brief description of contents. The medicine section comprises one-half of the June 1980 Quarterly Update. Films that may be rented are designated in this listing. A limited number of these titles may, as the issue indicates, be borrowed from the producing agency. Each issue includes audiovisuals in the following subjects: alcohol and drug abuse, business/government management, career education, consumer education, dentistry, education, emergency medical services, engineering, fire/law enforcement, flight/meteorology, health, history, industrial safety, medicine, science, social issues, social science, vocational education, and all aspects on new topics.
ENTRIES	Title (under subject), running time or number of frames, format, sound or silent, color or b/w, year of release, producer, title number, sale price, annotation, TV clearance, language (if other than English), special notes to users.
SPECIAL FEATURES	Includes information on additional services available from the National Audiovisual Center, title index, a section on withdrawn titles, and loan referrals.
ORDERING INFORMATION	Available from The National Audiovisual Center.
PRICE	Free.

RADIOLOGICAL HEALTH TRAINING RESOURCES CATALOG 1981

Bureau of Radiological Health, Food and Drug Administration, Public Health Service. U.S. Department of Health, Education, and Welfare. August 1981. 41 p. Prepared by Kaye F. Chesemore.

MEDIA	16mm films, videocassettes, audiocassettes.
SUMMARY	This catalog includes approximately 230 audiovisual programs produced by the Bureau of Radiological Health (BRH) for use by Federal, State, and local governments, industry, hospitals, the medical profession, educators, researchers, libraries, professional and trade organizations, the press, and others. These programs are also made available to the World Health Organization (WHO), for a world-wide distribution. WHO, at times, participates in the development of these programs. The audiovisuals included in this catalog are limited to radiological health subjects only. They represent a variety of topics ranging from basic fundamentals to historical perspectives to current state of the art. The materials are classified by subject area listed under the following headings: basic principles of radiation detection, basic theory of radiation protection, beneficial applications of radiation, biological effects of radiation, factors affecting radiographic images and patient exposure, fundamentals of radiation emitting machines, non-ionizing radiation, nuclear medicine, protection from radiation emitting machines, protection from radioactive materials, radiation inspections and surveys, radiation interactions with matter, radiation therapy, miscellaneous. In the last category are included vignettes of early radiation workers featuring various scientists in the field of radiology expressing their experience and research produced between 1977-1980. The work of prominent scientists, interviews with them, the activities of the Nuclear Regulatory Commission during the Three Mile Island accident, the work of the World Health Organization (WHO), and similar scientific works are included in these audiovisuals. The entries are current but a few considered of historical value produced since 1950 are also included.
ENTRIES	Accession number, title, author responsible for the content, running time, color or b/w, evaluation, year of release.
SPECIAL FEATURES	Includes information on the activities of the Bureau of Radiological Health, list of materials available from other sources, listing of regional radiological health representatives, and request for borrowing forms.
ORDERING INFORMATION	Available from the Bureau of Radiological Health, Department of Health and Human Services. HHS Publication FDA 81-8023.
PRICE	Free from the Bureau of Radiological Health.

RECENT FILM RELEASES of the U.S. DEPARTMENT of AGRICULTURE

Office of Communications. U.S. Department of Agriculture. [1974]. [10] p. (Loose-leaf.)

MEDIA	16mm films, filmstrips, slide sets.
SUMMARY	Includes 30 color audiovisuals exclusively available through the film libraries of the various State Land Grant Universities included in their perspective catalogs. A list of these libraries is included in this release. Broad Subject categories included are: agriculture, climate, communicable diseases, entomology, environmental sciences, epidemiology, foreign language, government programs, poisoning, recreation, research, societies, space sciences, standards and statistics, wildlife, world health. These audiovisuals have been produced within the last ten years and have received numerous honors and awards. For a more complete listing of subjects see *BIMONTHLY LIST of PUBLICATIONS and AUDIOVISUALS* (located in every library), and *STATE FILMS CATALOGS on AGRICULTURE* included in this publication. Sample of state publications for Audiovisuals is included in this book (see *FILM LOAN SERVICE*, Minnesota Department of Natural Resources).
ENTRIES	Title, color, TV clearance, annotation, year of release (when available), awards.
SPECIAL FEATURES	Includes names and addresses of 51 State Land Grant University Libraries.
ORDERING INFORMATION	Available from the U.S. Department of Agriculture.
PRICE	Free.

REFERENCE LIST of AUDIOVISUAL MATERIALS PRODUCED by the UNITED STATES GOVERNMENT*

National Audiovisual Center, National Archives and Records Service. U.S. General Services Administration. 1978. 388 p. Supplement 1980. 90 p. Plus announcements and special subjects catalogs. (See summary below.)

MEDIA 16mm films, videocassettes, slide sets, audiotapes, multimedia kits. (16mm films are also available in ¾" videocassette format and videotape.)

SUMMARY This catalog lists over 7,000 audiovisual materials selected from over 15,000 programs produced by 175 Federal agencies since 1900, covering a wide variety of subjects. Major subject concentrations in the Center's collection include medicine, dentistry and allied health, education, science, social studies, industrial/technical training, and environmental sciences. The audiovisuals included in this publication are classified under the following broad subject headings: agriculture, arthritis, atomic energy, aviation, biology, business and economics, chemistry, civics and government, dentistry, drugs, education, electricity, electronics, engineering, eye, geography, health, history, humanities, hypertension, industrial arts, marine, medicine, mental health, military science, nursing, poisoning, physical science, sociology, space programs, surgery. Non-current audiovisuals considered of historical value are included for those engaged in research or interested in the history of subjects included in this catalog. Since 1977 the Center has been publishing a selected listings of U.S. Government audiovisuals appropriate for academic and professional education in various subjects. The following listings are: Alcohol and Drug problems, Business and Government Management, Career Education, Consumer Education, Dentistry, Documentary, Drug Abuse Prevention, Emergency Medical Services, Environment and Energy Conservation, Fire and Law Enforcement, Flight and Meteorology, Foreign Language Instruction, History, Industrial Safety, Library and Information Science, Medicine, Nursing, Social Issues, Spanish Language Soundtracks, Special Education, and Vocational Education. (See individual titles.)

SUPPLEMENT 1980. 90 p.

SUMMARY Lists over 1,000 new audiovisuals produced since 1978 by Federal agencies. The Major Subject List of the *Reference List 1978* edition (see above) is expanded and includes anthropology, fine arts, forestry, language, natural resources, and naval sciences. New specific subjects included are: air traffic control, arts (fine arts, crafts, museums), chemical and biological warfare, dentistry (study and teaching), energy (general), forensic medicine, health-related occupations, industrial hygiene, languages (Arabic, Baluchi, English), naval sciences (general), parent-child relationships, religion, safety (equipment, security planning), social ethics, and history of the space program. The Center serves as a central information clearinghouse for government-produced media. Its distribution program includes sales, loans, and rentals to both government agencies and to the public. For information on catalogs, brochures, and lists write to: National Archives and Records Service, Reference Section R.L., Washington, D.C. 20409. (301) 763-1896.

ENTRIES
Title, running time or number of frames, format, sound or silent, color or b/w, year of release, producer/sponsor, title number, rental or sale information, annotation, accompanying print material(s), series, additional notes on use or production, and, for medical and technical entries the educational author(s).

SPECIAL FEATURES
Includes an outline of subject headings, sponsor/producer codes, rental and purchase policies, price list.

ORDERING INFORMATION
Available from the Superintendent of Documents. U.S. Government Printing Office. Stock Number 052-003-00497-6. Suppl. 022-002-00069-4.

PRICE
1978 edition—$8.00; 1980 supplement—$4.25. All special subject supplements are free of charge from the National Audiovisual Center.

The RESOURCE FILE: PRACTICAL PUBLICATIONS for ENERGY MANAGEMENT. *A Reference Guide to Handbooks, Curricula, and Audiovisual Materials.*

United States Department of Energy. March 1978. [280] p. In various pagings.

(Prepared by JRB Associates, Inc., for the Assistant Secretary for Conservation and Solar Applications Under Contract No. EL-76-C-01-8656.)

MEDIA	16mm, 35mm films, filmstrips, videocassettes, slide sets, audiocassettes.
SUMMARY	This publication includes both print and audiovisual materials produced and/or published by both government and independent producers. It is a reference tool, designed for anyone who is asked to recommend "how-to" conservation guides to the public, or who wishes to select one for himself. Managers, facility engineers, building owners and operators, staff development coordinators, consumer affairs professionals, architects, educators, extension agencies, librarians, all those involved in health and environmental sciences, and technical information specialists are among those who will find this guide useful. The publication is divided in the following major categories: agricultural facilities and operations, commercial establishments; office buildings, general materials that are applicable to the number of different topic areas, industrial plants and processes; power generation, residential; health care institutions, other housing, transportation; mobile equipment, films; filmstrips; videocassettes, supplementary resources. The 20 audiovisuals produced by both government agencies and independent producers cover the following specific subjects: climatology related to energy, community services, conservation (all aspects), consumer education about energy, energy engineering (including safety), energy for hospitals, environmental sciences, various heating systems, transportation. Many audiovisuals are available to the public on a free-loan basis from the United States Department of Energy. All entries are produced since 1974 and later.
ENTRIES	Title, producing government agency/producer, year of release, annotation, audience target recommendations, running time or number of frames, color or b/w, sound or silent, format, accompanying print materials and prices, audiovisual prices, availability/distribution information, distributor other than the government agency.
SPECIAL FEATURES	Includes an in-depth annotated bibliography of nonprint materials related to audiovisuals, a list of other Department of Energy (DOE) publications, and title and key word indexes. Order forms are also included.

ORDERING INFORMATION Available from the Superintendent of Documents, U.S. Government Printing Office. Stock No. 061-000-00049-6.

PRICE $5.50.

RESOURCES in WOMEN'S EDUCATIONAL EQUITY NON-PRINT MEDIA and MATERIALS

Office of Education. U.S. Department of Health, Education, and Welfare (Education Division). February 1978. 243 p.

MEDIA	16mm films, filmstrips, videocassettes, audiotapes, recordings.
SUMMARY	This publication includes 310 audiovisuals and some educational guides. Broad subject categories are: bibliographies, biographies, and portraits of women, family and life styles, history of women, laws and legislation (equal rights), sex roles and stereotypes, women and work. Specific subjects covered are: birth control and family planning, biological sciences, child care, counseling, history of women in medicine, hospital care, mental health, nursing, occupational diseases, physical fitness, rape, suicide. Many items are translated into the Braille system for use by the visually handicapped. The catalog is divided into the following sections: selected resources of non-print media and materials, items not classified, title index, audience type index, and list of distributors.
ENTRIES	Title, letter assigned to subject area, number which designates its order within the subject area, NICEM (National Information Center Media) and NIMIS (National Instructional Materials Information System) designated numbers, author, distributor, format, running time or number of frames, color or b/w, audience level, sale price, annotation, source.
SPECIAL FEATURES	The 1974 Women's Educational Equity Act is explained and the functions of the Women's Educational Equity Communications Network is presented. Title index and a list of distributors are included. (See summary also.)
ORDERING INFORMATION	Available from the Superintendent of Documents, U.S. Government Printing Office: Stock Number 017-080-01836-5. (Prepared by the Educational Testing Service, Princeton, New Jersey. Contract number 300-76-04-63 with the Office of Education, U.S. Department of Health, Education, and Welfare under the auspices of the Women's Educational Equity Act.)
PRICE	$9.95.

SELECTED AUDIOVISUALS on MENTAL HEALTH

National Institute of Mental Health, Alcohol, Drug Abuse, and Mental Health Administration. U.S. Department of Health, Education, and Welfare. 1975. 223 p.

MEDIA	16mm films, filmstrips, videocassettes.
SUMMARY	Contains approximately 2,300 entries of audiovisual materials produced by both U.S. Government agencies and commercial producers in the field of mental illness and mental health. These audiovisuals are available to persons engaged in educating the public and scientific audiences about mental illness and mental health. Subjects include: aging, animal studies, biochemistry and metabolism, child mental health, cognition and perception, communication, community mental health, crime and delinquency, cultural studies, death and suicide, depression, education, family, group processes, learning, mental retardation, minority groups, motivation, neurosciences, personality, psychology, religion, schizophrenia, sexology, sleep and dreams, social issues, treatment.
ENTRIES	Accession number, producer, distributor, rental or sale price, running time, color of b/w, year of release, annotation.
SPECIAL FEATURES	Includes sources for free loan welfare films, sources for low-cost film rental, commercial rental libraries, and complete rental information.
ORDERING INFORMATION	Available from the Superintendent of Documents, U.S. Government Printing Office: 176 0-202-710.
PRICE	$7.00.

SELECTED EDUCATIONAL MEDIA

West Point. U.S. Military Academy Library. 1977. 116 p. (1972- .)

MEDIA	16mm films, filmstrips, videocassettes, slide sets, recordings, still photographs.
SUMMARY	This listing provides a subject approach to the wide variety of non-book educational media held in the room of the USMA (United States Military Academy) library. Materials are listed under the following major subjects: alcohol and alcoholism, biology, chemistry, drug abuse, earth sciences, ecology, energy, food, general sciences, geology, natural disaster, pollution, space sciences, urban studies. warfare.
ENTRIES	Title, framed art prints, running time or number of frames, format, color or b/w, sound or silent, audience.
SPECIAL FEATURES	This publication is in machine-readable form for on-line searching and is updated annually. Restricted borrowing privileges.
ORDERING INFORMATION	Available from the National Technical Information Service (NTIS).
PRICE	Not available (NTIS).

SELECTED FILMS: HEART DISEASE, CANCER, and STROKE

Public Health Service Audiovisual Facility, Communicable Disease Center[1], Bureau of Disease Prevention and Environmental Control, U.S. Department of Health, Education, and Welfare, Public Health Service. January 1968. 96 p.

MEDIA
16mm films.

SUMMARY
Approximately 150 films on heart diseases, cancer, and stroke professionally selected from the files of the *International Index of Medical Film Data*[2], located in the Public Health Service Audiovisual Facility (presently in the National Medical Audiovisual Center (NMAC). Most of them are films of the American Heart Association, and the American Cancer Society. The films provide a broad coverage of information, research, and treatment in the three medical areas: heart disease, cancer, and stroke. Films in pioneer work of prominent heart and cancer specialists are also included in this brochure. The catalog is divided in three sections: heart disease, cancer, and stroke. Each section is further divided into professional and nonprofessional films.

ENTRIES
Title, producer, author (if available), year of release, edition, country of origin, running time, sound or silent, color or b/w, format, annotation, distributor, distributor's identification number.

SPECIAL FEATURES
Includes information on the selection process of the films. A list of distributors is also included.

ORDERING INFORMATION
Available from the National Medical Audiovisual Center (NMAC). Complimentary copy from Public Health Service Publication No. 1780.

PRICE
Free.

---

[1] The audiovisual facility of the Public Health Service in Atlanta, Georgia, was transferred to NLM (National Library of Medicine) from the National Communicable Disease Center and redesignated the National Medical Audiovisual Center (NMAC). Grove, Pearce S., and Clement, Evelyn G., eds. *Bibliographic Control of Nonprint Media.* Chicago American Library Association, 1972. p. 163-165.

[2] One of the world's largest collection of abstracts on medically related audiovisuals. It contains over 30,000 entries and was started after WWII at the National Library of Medicine (NLM), when it was known as the Armed Forces Medical Library. Grove. op. cit., p. 164.

A SELECTED GUIDE to AUDIO-VISUAL MATERIALS on ALCOHOL and ALCOHOLISM

National Clearinghouse for Alcohol Information, National Institute on Alcohol Abuse and Alcoholism, Public Health Service, Alcohol, Drug Abuse, and Mental Health Administration. U.S. Department of Health, Education, and Welfare. [1975]. 36 p.

MEDIA	16mm films.
SUMMARY	Contains approximately 260 films, television announcements, and radio announcements and programs classified under 60 categories. These programs are available from government agencies and commercial distributors, and cover approximately 60 subject areas. Films listed have been selected from many educational films produced since 1960 on the topics of alcohol and its misuse. The catalog is divided into 5 sections: films, which include a synopsis of content; additional films, which give titles and distributors; television announcements, radio spots, and scripts available from the National Institute on Alcohol Abuse and Alcoholism; and radio programs, with 28 3-minute radio programs available from commercial sponsors.
ENTRIES	Title, year of release, TV clearance, running time, color or b/w, intendent audience, sale or rental price, distributor, annotation.
SPECIAL FEATURES	Includes a list of additional films, TV announcements, radio programs, additional resources (film guides, public information programs, The National Clearinghouse for Alcohol Information activities and services), order form. A general subject index is also included.
ORDERING INFORMATION	Available from the Superintendent of Documents, U.S. Government Printing Office: 1975-0-591-923.
PRICE	Free.

SELECTED LIST: ALCOHOL and DRUG PROBLEMS

National Audiovisual Center, National Archives and Records Service. U.S. General Services Administration. 1981. 13 p.

MEDIA	16mm films, videotapes, audiotapes, multimedia kits, recordings.
SUMMARY	Includes approximately 50 audiovisual programs covering amphetamines, community action, depressants, drug culture, drug education, drug research, drug use, hallucinogens, heroin, opium, pharmacology and drugs, and speed. The catalog is divided into the following sections: alcohol and the body; alcohol and youth; alcohol—counseling and rehabilitation; drugs and the body; drugs—counseling and rehabilitation; tobacco. All materials are produced by various U.S. Government agencies and are available for rent or purchase from the National Audiovisual Center.
ENTRIES	Title, running time or number of frames, color or b/w, year of release, format, producing agency, title number, annotation, series identification, availability.
SPECIAL FEATURES	Gives information on other catalogs published by the National Audiovisual Center, ordering information, and information on public services provided by the Center. Title index is also included.
ORDERING INFORMATION	Available from The National Audiovisual Center.
PRICE	Free.

SMITHSONIAN SLIDE SERIES. SLIDES. FILMSTRIPS. AUDIOCASSETTES. BOOKLETS.

Photographic Services. Smithsonian Institution. (Loose-leaf.) Current.

(The Smithsonian Institution has no single complete catalog of all Audiovisual materials available for sale. Requests are researched through specific division of the Institution responsible for each specific topical material. Photographs with annotations describing a subject, and a list of subjects under specific division are available.)

MEDIA	Filmstrips, slide sets, audiocassettes, transparencies.
SUMMARY	Loose-leaf package containing 20 pictorial entries and a list of general subjects under specific topical material. Medicine and allied health subjects included are: *Museum of Natural History* (MNH): animals, anthropology, athropods, entomology, evolution, zoology. *Museum of American History* (MAH): medical sciences, nuclear energy, old world archeology, physical sciences, photography, satellites (Einstein), technology, transportation. *National Air and Space Museum* (NASM): air transportation, aviation, sea-air operations, history of flight, skylab. These materials represent the past, present, and research for the future.
ENTRIES	[Entries courtesy of the Smithsonian Institution] : picture, title, note on subject, annotation, format, number of frames, language, accompanying print and pictorial material, additional print material such as bibliographies and articles, audience, availability. Price list is included in a separate sheet. In the list of categories identification number and title are given. ([Entries courtesy of the Smithsonian Institution] under special granted request.)
SPECIAL FEATURES	Includes guidelines for placing requests, what is available (format), how a subject is researched, information on reproduction of items. A price list is also included.
ORDERING INFORMATION	This brochure is available from the Customer Service Branch, Office of Printing and Photographic Services, Smithsonian Institution, Washington, D.C. 20560.
PRICE	Free.

SOURCE BOOK of EDUCATIONAL MATERIALS for RADIATION THERAPY

Bureau of Radiological Health, Food and Drug Administration, Public Health Service. U.S. Department of Health, Education, and Welfare. August 1981. 141 p. In various pagings. Prepared by Mary Lou Pijar and Jeannine T. Lewis.

MEDIA	16mm, 35mm films, filmstrips, videocassettes, slide sets, audiocassettes.
SUMMARY	This publication is divided into 22 sections, each section corresponding to a subject area included in the *Syllabus for Radiation Therapy Technology Education,* developed by the American Society of Radiologic Technologists. Each section is subdivided into subsections entitled Publications, and (within chapters) Audiovisuals and Training Aids. It includes both print and audiovisual materials of special interest to individuals involved in radiation therapy. The 272 audiovisuals, most of them current, cover the following specific subjects: anatomy and physiology, biological effects of ionizing radiation and protection, blood (collection), CPR (cardiopulmonary resuscitation), chemistry, clergy in cancer management (family and patient counseling), chromatography, communicable diseases (V.D.), communications (interpersonal communications series), computers, death (family counseling), endocrinology, epilepsy, first aid, genetics, jurisprudence/ethics, laboratory safety, language (non-English speaking patient), management, medical terminology, metric system, neoplasms (cancer/oncology), nuclear medicine (general), nursing, patient education, pediatrics, physics (radiologic), tomography (radiologic). The work of WHO (World Health Organization) and other scientific works are included in these audiovisuals. These audiovisuals are produced by both government agencies and independent producers and are available to the public on a free-loan basis from the Bureau of Radiological Health Training Resource Center. They are also made available to WHO for world-wide distribution.
ENTRIES	Title, author responsible for the content and his professional affiliation(s), producer, format, running time, year of release, distributor, ordering number, annotation, additional notes, rental and purchase prices for materials available from commercial agencies.
SPECIAL FEATURES	Includes information on the activities of the Bureau of Radiological Health, directory of sources, a list of audiovisual producers, a list of related periodicals (by independent publishers), and list of publications published by the Bureau of Radiological Health (BRH) available to the public from the U.S. Government Printing Office.

ORDERING INFORMATION	Available from the Superintendent of Documents, U.S. Government Printing Office: HHS Publication FDA 80-8157.
PRICE	$5.50. Single copy available free of charge from the Bureau of Radiological Health.

SPACE BENEFITS: NASA FILMS and PUBLICATIONS DESCRIBING BENEFITS of SPACE and TECHNOLOGY

U.S. National Aeronautics and Space Administration. 1976. 10 p.

MEDIA	16mm films, filmstrips, audiotapes.
SUMMARY	This publication includes both print and nonprint materials published and produced by the National Aeronautics and Space Administration designed to meet the needs of educators, students, and the general public. They describe and explain in everyday terms NASA's aerospace activities, advances in science and engineering resulting from NASA programs, and how aerospace technology is being adapted to benefit people on earth. Subjects covered by both print and nonprint materials are: application of satellites in medicine and agriculture, computer programs (NASTRAN) for solving problems in industry, earth resources, first aid in natural disasters, NASA's research in health sciences, oceanography, parametics, pollution, space laboratory. The 20 nonprint materials have received many awards in the United States and abroad. They are available for showing free of charge for U.S. citizens through the NASA Regional Libraries, and in foreign countries through the Pacific Affairs Officer, U.S. Information Service at the American Embassy in their National Capital. The catalog is divided into the following sections: filmstrips, films, rediscovery series, NASA audiotapes, educational and special interest films, educational publications NASA facts.
ENTRIES	Title, ordering number, year of release, color or b/w, running time or number of frames, annotation, awards, related items within the catalog.
SPECIAL FEATURES	Includes a list of NASA Regional Film Libraries, information on loan or purchase of print and nonprint materials, film prices, education publications concerned with space science.
ORDERING INFORMATION	Available from the Superintendent of Documents, U.S. Government Printing Office: GPO:1976–206-280. (Price not available.)
PRICE	Single copy free from NASA.

SPECIAL EDUCATION: SELECTED U.S. GOVERNMENT AUDIOVISUALS

National Audiovisual Center, National Archives and Records Service. U.S. General Services Administration. October 1977. 61 p.

MEDIA	16mm films, filmstrips, videocassettes, slide sets, audiotapes, multimedia kits, transparencies, recordings. Indexes (Locaters) are also included.
SUMMARY	Contains approximately 150 audiovisual materials selected from the 13,000 titles of the computer data files of the National Audiovisual Center's collections. These materials are for teaching and training of the hearing impaired, deaf, handicapped children, multiply handicapped, mentally retarded, and those with learning disabilities. These materials are available from the Center for use by schools, librarians, institutions, industry, and the general public.
ENTRIES	Title, running time, format, optical, sound or silent, color or b/w, year of release, title numbers, sale price, annotation, TV clearance, series, additional notes on use of production. (See also *Catalog of Educational Captioned Films for the Deaf 1980-81.*)
SPECIAL FEATURES	Includes information on other catalogs published by the Center, ordering information, information on other public services by the Center. The catalog is divided into subject sections. Includes bibliographies other than Audiovisuals.
ORDERING INFORMATION	Available from The National Audiovisual Center.
PRICE	Free.

35 ENERGY FILMS

U.S. Department of Energy. 1981. 21 p.

(For a complete listing of films available from the U.S. Department of Energy see ENERGY FILMS CATALOG.)

SUMMARY	This catalog includes 35 current films produced by U.S. Government agencies or by independent producers for the Department of Energy (DOE). These films are available on a free-loan basis to educational, civic, library, television, industrial, professional youth activity, and government organizations. Subjects covered are: agriculture, alternative sources to energy, coal, cooling water systems, electric power, energy conservation, energy management, environmental sciences, gasohol, geothermal energy, home energy, natural energy, history and future of energy, nuclear weapons (Nevada Test Site), oil, transportation, wind energy. Many of these films have received numerous national and international awards.
ENTRIES	Film number, title, running time, color or b/w, audience level, annotation, year of release, producer, sale source, TV clearance, awards.
SPECIAL FEATURES	Includes loan information, TV clearance, copyright, video copying, information on how to obtain film footage, civil rights, request forms. Title index is also included.
ORDERING INFORMATION	Available from DOE Film Library.
PRICE	Free.

TRAINING FILMS [Mine Safety and Health Administration (MSHA)] 1981-1982

Mine Safety and Health Administration. U.S. Department of Labor. 1981. 33 p.

MEDIA	16mm films. (Only videocassette format for purchase).
SUMMARY	This catalog included 65 films produced by the MSHA (Mine Safety and Health Administration) as a part of a nationwide effort to improve the health and safety of mining personnel. All films are available for loan to the mineral industries, educational institutions, engineering and scientific societies, business and civic clubs, fraternal groups, and other responsible organizations in the United States. The films are also available internationally for purchase only. The entries are classified under the broad subject categories: Coal mining, Metal and Non-metal Mining, Coal and Metal and Nonmetal Mining, and First Aid. Specific subjects covered are: accidents and their prevention, emergencies, environmental sciences, equipment design and safety, first aid, jurisprudence, laboratory, occupational and preventive medicine, public health, radiation (handling and safety), safety (general), transportation. Most of the films are current but some date back to 1960. Many entries have received national and international awards.
ENTRIES	Film number, title, edition, year of release, running time, annotation, awards.
SPECIAL FEATURES	Includes a list of award winning films, general information on borrowing or purchase films, subject index, TV clearance, price list, and order form. A title index listing films under broad categories is also included.
ORDERING INFORMATION	Available from MSHA Office.
PRICE	Free.

UNION LIST of AUDIOVISUALS in the LIBRARY NETWORK of the VETERANS ADMINISTRATION*

Library Division, Learning Resources Service, Office of Academic Affairs, Department of Medicine and Surgery. U.S. Veterans Administration. September 1976. 595 p.

MEDIA	16mm films, videocassettes, slide sets, audiocassettes.
SUMMARY	This listing contains approximately 3,500 entries of audiovisual materials produced by both U.S. Government agencies and independent producers. This comprehensive listing covers all aspects in medicine and allied health. The subject reading authority section lists 1,680 subject headings. Broad subject categories covered are: accident and accident prevention, alcohol and alcoholism, anatomy and histology, anesthesiology, arthritis, biology, body as a whole, cancer, cardiovascular system, chemistry, child abuse, child development, cytology and tissue culture, dentistry, dermatology, digestive system, drugs and therapeutics, embryology, emergency health services, environmental (social) and environmental health, epilepsy, eye, first aid, food, forensic medicine, genetics, geriatrics, health education, hematology, hospital administration, hypertension, hypnosis, Indians (North American), infectious diseases, microbiology, minority groups, musculoskeletal system, nursing and patient care, otorhinolargyngology, pediatrics, pharmacology and pharmacognosy, physical fitness, physiology, preventive medicine, psychiatry and psychology, public health, radiology, reconstructive surgery, rehabilitation, respiratory system, sex education, social sciences, surgery, technology (medical), thanatology, toxicology, urogenital system, veterinary medicine, vocational guidance, volunteer work, yoga. These audiovisual materials are available to the public free of charge through the 138 Veterans Administration Libraries in the Network around the country listed in the catalog. (See also *Dental Training Films* and *VA Film Catalog.*)
ENTRIES	Title, author(s) and his (their) affiliation or producer, year of release, running time or number of frames, format, accompanying print material(s), audience level, sound or silent, color or b/w, annotation, subject(s), ordering information, item number for identification purposes.
SPECIAL FEATURES	This union list may be used to identify entries by author, title, and subject, since author and subject indexes are included. A list of the 138 Veterans Administration Libraries in the Network is given in a separate supplement.

ORDERING INFORMATION   Available from the Superintendent of Documents, U.S. Government Printing Office: 1976 0-240-992(506).

PRICE $16.50.

UNITED STATES GOVERNMENT MOTION PICTURES and TELEVISION PROGRAMS SUBMITTED in 1980 and 1981 to INTERNATIONAL FILM and TELEVISION EVENTS

Interdepartmental Subcommittee on Selection of Motion Pictures. U.S. International Communication Agency. 1981, 20 p. 1981, 21 p.

MEDIA	Motion pictures, filmstrips, slide sets, recordings models, maps, charts, posters, and other audiovisual materials.
SUMMARY	1980 list: includes entries shown in 1980 festivals in the United States, Canada, Europe, and other continents. These films are produced by the United States Government Agencies and cover liberal arts and sciences, medical and allied health. Some of these materials are available from the National Audiovisual Center, National Archives and Records Service, U.S. General Services Administration. 1981 list: This is a working document prepared by the International Communications Media Division, Television Film Service, International Communication Agency, listing, when known, scheduled events for film and television events to be held in 1981-1982. Information included is: country, city, number of festival (year), month, date, year. (Listing of specific subjects and titles are not available at the present. *General Information.* The International Communication Agency (ICA) administers for the United States the multilateral treaty, Agreement for Facilitating the International Circulation of Visual and Auditory Materials of an Education, Scientific and Cultural Character (Beirut Agreement of 1948). Under this agreement a number of countries permit the duty-free importations of audiovisual materials, and freedom from certain non-tariff restrictions. U.S. producers and sponsors of audiovisual materials participate under an agreement with the International Communication Agency. For more information write to: Attention Office of the United States (PGM/T) International Communication Agency, 1776 Pennsylvania Avenue, N.W., Washington, D.C. 20547. Telephone (202) 376-7203.
ORDERING INFORMATION	Available from the International Communications Agency.
PRICE	Free.

VA FILM CATALOG

U.S. Veterans Administration. January 1980. 100 p.

MEDIA	16mm films, filmstrips, videocassettes, slide sets, audiocassettes.
SUMMARY	This catalog lists over 700 audiovisual materials produced by the U.S. Government and by independent producers for the Veterans Administration since 1950. These audiovisuals are available on a free-loan basis from the Veterans Administration Office Film Library, and are designed to support medical and scientific research programs and studies, and for orientation, training, and information. The catalog is divided in major subject sections, and under each section entries of specific subjects are listed: Chaplain Service (for use only by the Veterans Administration Chaplain Service); Dentistry: anatomy and physiology, complete dentures, dental assisting, diagnosis, endodontics, esthetics, fixed partial dentures, materials, occlusion, operative dentistry, oral hygiene and patient education, periodontics, prosthodontics, radiology (oral), removable partial dentures, surgery (oral). Health: dietetics, drug abuse and alcoholism, public health, sanitation. Medicine: cardiovascular system, gastrointestinal system, hemic and lymphatic systems, hospital administration, infectious disease, musculoskeletal system, nervous system, nursing and home care, practice of medicine, respiratory system. Personnel training: career recruitment, food preparation and handling, human relations, job training, management and supervision. Psychiatry and Psychology. Rehabiliation: geriatrics, occupation and physical therapy. Safety: accident prevention, hospital safety. Surgery. Veterans Administration: services and special ceremonies. Miscellaneous: clergy, death in the battlefield, handicapped, physical fitness, radioisotopes. (See also *Dental Training Films* and *Union List of Audiovisuals in the Library Network of the Veterans Administration.*)
ENTRIES	Title, running time or number of frames, format, sound or silent, color or b/w, producer, author (when available), title numbers, annotation, accompanying print material(s).
SPECIAL FEATURES	Includes information on other services by the Veterans Administration, ordering information, outline of subject and sub-topic headings, subject index, and title index.
ORDERING INFORMATION	Available from the Superintendent of Documents, U.S. Government Printing Office: Stock Number 051-000-00138-9.
PRICE	$4.25.

VENEREAL DISEASE FILMS (For the General Public)

Center for Disease Control, Public Health Service. U.S. Department of Health, Education, and Welfare. 1974. 16 p.

MEDIA	16mm films, super-8 cassettes, videocassettes.
SUMMARY	Includes 25 audiovisual entries on venereal diseases for general public use. These audiovisuals are available from the State Departments of Health, from commercial distributors, pharmaceutical companies, from university centers, or the National Audiovisual Center (NAC). Subjects covered are: cases of the disease, history of medical knowledge, "Operation Venus" (hotline information center), patient education, prophylaxis, sex education for parents and children, treatment. Some audiovisuals are available in French, Spanish, German, Italian, and Swedish languages. Many TV and motion picture celebrities appear in the programs. Most of the entries are current but some date back to 1950.
ENTRIES	Title, running time, color or b/w, sound or silent, year of release, TV clearance, annotation, accompanying print material, rental and sale source(s), language.
SPECIAL FEATURES	Provides full rental and purchase information giving more than one source.
ORDERING INFORMATION	Available from the Center of Disease Control. Publication No. 9F0946574.
PRICE	Free.

VIDEO TAPE CATALOG CONTINUING MEDICAL EDUCATION and INSTRUCTION

Academy of Health Sciences. United States Army (AHSUSA). 9th edition. Fort Sam Houston, Texas. 1981. (Loose-leaf). Plus supplements.

MEDIA	Videocassettes.
SUMMARY	Contains annotated entries for approximately 1,000 highly technical videocassettes produced since 1968 and intended for those concerned with education of medical students, interns, residents, physicians in all specialties, and those in fields allied with medicine. Subject areas include: behavioral sciences, cardiovascular system, dentistry, dermatology, drug abuse, gynecology, internal medicine, nursing, otorhinolaryngology, pharmacology, psychiatry and psychology, surgery, veterinary medicine. The catalog is divided into two sections: Continuing Education Programs, and Medical Training and Instruction Programs. Each section is further divided into a numerical index of program titles, an index of programs under supporting departments, and videotape data sheets in numerical order describing the content of programs.
ENTRIES	Videocassette number, clearance category number, title, annotation, year of release, running time, lesson plan number, objectives, target audience, remarks (recording specifications), person(s) responsible for the content (author(s)/cosponsor(s)), and their affiliation, including address.
SPECIAL FEATURES	Includes ordering information and procedures instructions indicating that free copying of programs is available to non-profit medical agencies upon request. (Sufficient blank videotape must be provided. This three-ring binder is easy to upgrade by inserting supplemental sheets indicating new and deleted entries.) Title index is provided for each section.
ORDERING INFORMATION	Available from the U.S. Department of the Army, Academy of Health Sciences, Fort Sam Houston, Texas. C, Health Sciences Media Division, AHS. Publication No. (HSA-ZHD 900334).
PRICE	$7.00.

VIKING FILM ANNOUNCEMENT

U.S. National Aeronautics and Space Administration, Office of Public Affairs. 1976. 6 p.

MEDIA	16mm films.
SUMMARY	Includes eight annotated entries for 16mm films (all in color with sound) concerning NASA's search for life on other planets. Topics covered by these films include the following: biomedical evidence of life, general characteristics of life as we know it, extraterrestrial life, excerpts from Orson Welles' 1938 radio broadcasts, "The War of the Worlds," hypothetical conclusions of types of possible life forms, and related life sciences areas.
ENTRIES	Title, ordering number, sound, color, running time, number and names of awards.
SPECIAL FEATURES	Includes an introduction on the Viking spacecraft program, pictures in various pages, a list of NASA Regional Film Libraries, and order form.
ORDERING INFORMATION	Available from NASA Office of Public Affairs. GPO:1976 0-599-782 (NASA-451).
PRICE	Free.

WHERE the DRUG FILMS ARE: A GUIDE to EVALUATION SERVICES and DISTRIBUTORS

National Institute on Drug Abuse, Alcohol, and Mental Health Administration, Public Health Service. U.S. Department of Health, Education, and Welfare. 1977. 19 p.

MEDIA	16mm films.
SUMMARY	This guide describes the drug film evaluation services in the United States and lists commercial distributors of drug films in this country. In addition, this source is designed to help the public locate inexpensive and convenient sources of films, sources for federal materials, and commercial and nonprofit distributors. The information included provides prices on sale and rental, the availability of preview prints, and the titles of the audiovisuals distributed by commercial firms, trade associations, government agencies, and religious organizations. All films listed are evaluated, and an alphabetical list of federal agencies is provided.
SPECIAL FEATURES	Includes lists of commercial and nonprofit distributors, future films, materials available from Federal agencies, and Federal agencies which are distributing inexpensive and convenient sources. Group of films handled by specific distributors is also included.
ORDERING INFORMATION	Free copy is provided by the Alcohol, Drug Abuse, and Mental Health Administration, Printing and Publications Management Section. DHEW Publication No. (ADM) 77-429.

Special Items

bibliographies
personnel/AV—Government
reports
state publications (samples)
others

AoA FACT SHEET: AUDIOVISUAL MATERIALS SPONSORED by the ADMINISTRATION on AGING

National Clearinghouse on Aging, Administration on Aging, Office of Human Development. U.S. Department of Health, Education, and Welfare. June 1981. (Irregular.)

MEDIA	16mm films, videocassettes.
SUMMARY	Includes announcements of new programs on gerontology produced by both government agencies and independent producers. Subjects cover all aspects on aging, both social and medical. It includes titles included in the National Audiovisual Center, universities, and in the International Center for Social Gerontology catalogs, availability and ordering information, prices, and duplicating restrictions. Film order form for rental and purchase of audiovisuals is also included. DHHS Publication No. (OHDS) 81-20031. For information on the AoA Fact Sheet write to: Human Development Services, National Clearinghouse on Aging, Administration on Aging, Washington, D.C. 20201. (See *AoA Catalog.*)
PRICE	Free from the Administration on Aging.

BRAILLE BOOK REVIEW

Publication Services, Division for the Blind and Physically Handicapped. U.S. Library of Congress. 1975- . Bimonthly.

MEDIA	Press Braille Books.
SUMMARY	This magazine informs readers on developments and activities for the blind and physically handicapped individuals. These materials are: newsstand items, press-braille books, hand-copied braille, braille magazines, letters from the users, new catalogs, and all new developments in the braille system. For a complete listing of subjects see: HEALTH: A SELECTED LIST of BOOKS that HAVE APPEARED in TALKING BOOK TOPICS AND BRAILLE BOOK TOPICS. *(See also Catalog of Educational Films for the Deaf 1980-81.)*
SPECIAL FEATURES	Includes information on how to use the system, eligibility, ordering information, surveys and studies, and related print materials. A subject/item index is included.
ORDERING INFORMATION	Available from the cooperating public library in the area. For additional information write to: Publication Services, Division for the Blind and Physically Handicapped, Library of Congress, Washington, D.C. 20542.
PRICE	Distributed free of charge to participants in the Library of Congress Braille Program.

DIRECTORY OF U.S. GOVERNMENT AUDIOVISUAL PERSONNEL

National Audiovisual Center, National Archives and Records Service. U.S. General Services Administration. 7th edition. 1980. 63 p.

SUMMARY | Published by the National Audiovisual Center this directory lists Federal agencies and their audiovisual personnel involved in television, motion pictures, still photography, sound recordings, and exhibits. It includes approximately 125 producing agencies, the names of their audiovisual personnel, addresses and phone numbers in the following branches: Legislative Branch, Judicial Branch, Executive Branch, Independent Establishments and Government Corporations, and Committees and Councils. It includes name and organization (agencies) indexes. An order form is also included. This directory can be used as a guideline for obtaining audiovisual catalogs or information on audiovisual activities conducted by the United States Government.

ORDERING INFORMATION | Available from the National Audiovisual Center.

PRICE | $5.00.

FILM CATALOG 1980. PACIFIC NORTHERN REGION.

U.S. Forest Service, Pacific Northwest Region. (Portland, Or.). 1980. 32 p.

(Included as a sample of the Pacific Northern Region audiovisual materials and services available within individual states.)

MEDIA	16mm films.
SUMMARY	This is a listing of 118 annotated films dealing with all aspects of agriculture, animal life, climate, conservation, fire prevention, forest product laboratory work, irrigation, man and the environment, natural resources, plant life, and wildlife. The catalog is divided into three parts: general interest films, which are available to the public; reserved films, which may be used by the general public (Forest Service representatives have first priority); and in-service training films, which are exclusively used by Forest Service personnel. NOTE: Some entries are included in the Eastern Region catalog.
ENTRIES	Title, running time, color or b/w, grade level, annotation, film library number, TV clearance.
SPECIAL FEATURES	Gives a list of states served by the Region.
ORDERING INFORMATION	Available from the Forest Service, U.S. Department of Agriculture, Pacific Northwest Region's Information Office, publication no. RG-10-014-1980.
PRICE	Free.

HEALTH: A SELECTED LIST of BOOKS that HAVE APPEARED in TALKING BOOK TOPICS and BRAILLE BOOK REVIEW

U.S. Library of Congress. National Library Service for the Blind and Physically Handicapped. 1979. [83] p.

MEDIA	Press Braille Books.
SUMMARY	Includes approximately 500 health science books translated into the Braille system to be used by the blind and those who are involved in programs for the blind and physically handicapped. Subjects covered are: aging, alcohol, arthritis, biography (patient–physicians–nurses), birth control, cancer, child care, diabetes, exercise, eyes, genetics, gynecology, heart and blood, hygiene, medical history and research, medicine, sleep and relaxation, surgery, therapeutics, venereal disease. Magazines and bibliographies related to those subjects are also listed. HEALTH is available in large print, Braille, and disc formats.
SPECIAL FEATURES	Includes information on how to use the system, eligibility, ordering information, and subscription form. Title index is also included.
ORDERING INFORMATION	Available from the cooperating public library in the area. For additional information write to: National Library Service for the Blind and Physically Handicapped, Library of Congress, Washington, D.C. 20542. (U.S. Government Printing Office: 1979-294-630.)
PRICE	Distributed free of charge to participants in the Library of Congress Braille Program.

MATERIALS from the NATIONAL ARTS and the HANDICAPPED INFORMATION SERVICE: ANNOTATED BIBLIOGRAPHY

National Endowment for the Humanities. 2nd draft. November 1978.

(This edition was supported in part by a grant from the American Telephone and Telegraph Company, and by a grant from the National Endowment for the Arts, Washington, D.C., a federal agency. November 1978.)

MEDIA	16mm films, recordings, materials transcribed in Braille format (books are also included).
SUMMARY	This annotated bibliography includes print and nonprint materials on the subject of arts for the handicapped persons produced since 1970. The names of five organizations that provide custom bibliographies of print and audiovisual materials are also included. This publication reviews instructional materials for the Library of Congress National Service for Blind and Physically Handicapped Braille. Includes the following sections: catalogs which are available from the Music Service Section, U.S. Library of Congress. Media: lists catalogs and films for loan, recent films about arts and the handicapped, recent videocassette programs about arts for the handicapped. Films for the deaf and hearing impaired. Captioned films. Where to write for listings of captioned films. Nonverbal films. Mixed Media. Materials are available for loan from the National Instructional Information System, cooperating network of 56 regional and more than 100 subregional or local resource centers/public libraries. The network was established by the Bureau of Education for the Handicapped. Each U.S. Office of Education Regional Resource Center provides free loan materials to its geographical area.
SPECIAL FEATURES	Includes information on Annual Film Festivals and their film listings and catalogs sponsored by the Children's Hospital of Los Angeles and the Association of Mental Disfunctions. Lists all films available and their 1976, 1977, and 1978 catalogs and their availability and cost. Gives information on how the materials included in the catalogs were collected. Includes a verified list of materials with a description abstracted from printed reviews and verifies availability. Bibliographies for those interested in books printed before 1970, press articles, reports, and dissertations are also listed.
ORDERING INFORMATION	Available from the National Technical Information (NTIS).
PRICE	$5.00. (Available also in microfiche.)

MEDICAL CINEMATOGRAPHY

National Medical Audiovisual Center, National Library of Medicine, Public Health Service. U.S. Department of Health, Education, and Welfare. 1979. 48 p.

MEDIA	Cinematographic illustrations.
SUMMARY	This three-part monograph describes and illustrates innovative specialized techniques for cinematography useful to those presently working in documenting needed information for teaching, research, and patient education, and also, to those creative individuals in seeking practical new application for improvement of the media in the health sciences and related scientific areas. Many photographs of cases and equipment used give information to all those engaged in documenting examinations (1) of the eye, (2) larynx, and (3) nasopharyx, or any of a wide range of procedures performed in the surgical suite.
SPECIAL FEATURES	Gives pictorial samples in black and white of specialized techniques used in the three areas (given in the summary), and includes a bibliography of entries dated back to 1883.
ORDERING INFORMATION	Available from the Superintendent of Documents, U.S. Government Printing Office Stock No. 017-023-00133-7. Publication No. 1979-0-644-944.
PRICE	$6.00.

MOTION PICTURES, FILMS, and AUDIOVISUAL INFORMATION: Subject Bibliography (Title varies)

United States Government Printing Office, Assistant Public Printer. (Superintendent of Documents. Various Issues. Looseleaf. Monthly publication. (Audiovisual section published irregularly.) [4] p.

MEDIA	Films, filmstrips, videocassettes, slide sets, audiotapes, multimedia kits, transparencies, recordings.
SUMMARY	This is a listing of the most recent audiovisual catalogs published by the U.S. Government and distributed by the U.S. Government Printing Office. Gives complete bibliographic information on catalogs and indexes, guides, handbooks, statistics, workshops, and meetings. For each entry title of publication, pages, L.C. and U.S. Government Printing Office ordering numbers, brief annotation of contents, format(s), and prices are given. Order form is also included.
ORDERING INFORMATION	Available from the Superintendent of Documents, U.S. Government Printing Office.
PRICE	Free.

NATURAL RESOURCES DEPARTMENT FILMS

Film Loan Service. Minnesota Department of Natural Resources, Bureau of Information and Education. [1981]. 22 p. (Included as a sample of State Film Services.)

(Included as a sample of Natural Resources audiovisual materials and services available within individual states.)

MEDIA	16mm films, slide sets.
SUMMARY	Includes approximately 600 audiovisual entries produced by the Natural Resources Department dealing with the environment. Specific subjects represented in these materials are: agriculture, bionomics, energy and conservation, firearms/safety and gun handling, food, forest fire and safety, irrigation, man's effects on the environment, natural disasters, sailing/safety, water resources/pollution. These films are available to any Minnesota organization. Those interested in environmental films should contact their State Conservation Departments.
ENTRIES	Title, running time, color or b/w, sound or silent, annotation.
SPECIAL FEATURES	Includes regulations for borrowing films, and a section on Environmental Educational Films.
ORDERING INFORMATION	Available from the Minnesota Department of Natural Resources.
PRICE	Free.

NMAC NEWS: SELECTED BIOMEDICAL AUDIOVISUALS

National Medical Audiovisual Center, National Library of Medicine, National Institutes of Health, Public Health Service. U.S. Department of Health, Education, and Welfare. July 1977. 42 p. Plus announcements.

(Programs are available for purchase from the National Audiovisual Center.)

MEDIA	16mm films, videocassettes, and slide sets.
SUMMARY	This is a complete listing of audiovisual materials sponsored by the National Medical Audiovisual Center (NMAC), National Library of Medicine, which are available for purchase from the National Audiovisual Center (NAC). NAC provides government agencies and the general public with central information, loan referrals, sales, and rental service for audiovisual materials produced by federal agencies.
ENTRIES	Titles are separated by media format. Title, title number, running time or number of frames, accompanying print or nonprint material(s), sound or silent, b/w, price (when for sale).
SPECIAL FEATURES	Includes information on how to purchase materials, and gives indexes of entries by media format.
ORDERING INFORMATION	Available from the National Medical Audiovisual Center (NMAC). U.S. Government Printing Office: 1977—740-100/803.
PRICE	Free.

PROBLEMS in BIBLIOGRAPHIC ACCESS to NON-PRINT MATERIALS, PROJECT MEDIA BASE: FINAL REPORT

National Commission on Libraries and Information Science. October 1979. 90 p.

SUMMARY	This report presents the Commission's conclusions and recommendations for the establishment of bibliographic control of audiovisual resources as a part of an overall objective to plan, develop, and implement a nationwide network of library and information services. The purpose of this project was to test the hypothesis that the essential elements of a national bibliographic system for audiovisual informational resources currently exist, and that therefore there is no apparent impediment to a national system. On the assumption that the hypothesis was correct, the project also sought to define function specifications for such an integrated system of audiovisual resources. Specific subjects covered are: audiovisual aids, information systems, audiovisual centers, cataloging, classification, libraries, library collections, library networks, and library programs. The Commission plans to continue its study.
ORDERING INFORMATION	Available from the Superintendent of Documents, U.S. Government Printing Office Stock Number 052-003-00714-2.
PRICE	$3.50.

TALKING BOOK TOPICS

Publication Services, Division for the Blind and Physically Handicapped. U.S. Library of Congress. 1975-. Bimonthly.

SUMMARY	This magazine informs readers of new developments and activities for the blind and physically handicapped individuals. The publication is divided according to standards of new topics such as newsstand, special reports, talking book records, talking books cassettes, books for adults, books for children, talking books magazines, new AV catalogs, discs, bestseller books, fiction and non-fiction. For a complete listing of subjects, see BRAILLE BOOK REVIEW, and TALKING BOOK TOPICS. The entire collection of talking books recorded in Spanish is listed in LIBROS PARLANTES edition. *(See also Catalog of Educational Films for the Deaf 1980-81.)*
ENTRIES	Title, author, narrator(s), identification number, annotation, year of publication.
SPECIAL FEATURES	Includes information on how to use the system, eligibility, ordering information, surveys and studies, and related print materials. A talking book magazine index is also included.
ORDERING INFORMATION	Available from the cooperating public library in the area. For additional information write to: Publication Services, Division for the Blind and Physically Handicapped, Library of Congress, Washington, D.C. 20542.
PRICE	Distributed free of charge to participants in the Library of Congress Talking Book Topics Program.

Agencies

For a complete listing of U.S. Government agencies, newly created, deleted agencies, or change of addresses, please consult the current edition of the U.S. GOVERNMENT AUDIOVISUAL PERSONNEL catalog published by the National Audiovisual Center (included in this book) or the U.S. GOVERNMENT ORGANIZATIONAL MANUAL.

Academy of the Health Sciences U.S. Army (AHSUSA)
Health Sciences Media Division, AHS
Fort Sam Houston, Texas 78234

Administration for Children, Youth, and Families
Department of Health, Education and Welfare
Washington, D.C. 20201

Administration on Aging
Department of Health, Education, and Welfare
Washington, D.C. 20201

Aerospace Audiovisual Service
Department of the Air Force
Washington, D.C. 20330

Agency for International Development (AID)
International Development Cooperation Agency, U.S.
Washington, D.C. 20523

Agriculture, Department of
Washington, D.C. 20250

Agriculture, Milwaukee, Wisconsin
Department of Agriculture
U.S. Forst Service. Eastern Section
c/o John Hall Films Service
Milwaukee, Wisconsin 53209

Agriculture, Portland, Oregon
Department of Agriculture
U.S. Forest Service. Pacific Northwest Region's Information Offices
Portland, Oregon 97208

Air Force, Department of the
Washington, D.C. 20330

Alcohol, Tobacco, and Firearms, Bureau of
Department of the Treasury
Washington, D.C. 20220

Alcohol, Drug Abuse, and Mental Health Administration
Public Health Service
200 Independence Avenue, SW
Washington, D.C. 20201

Animal and Plant Health Inspection
Department of Agriculture
Washington, D.C. 20250

Armed Forces Institute of Pathology
Department of Defense
Washington, D.C. 20306

Army Audiovisual Center
Department of the Army Headquarters
Room 5A470, Pentagon
Washington, D.C. 20310

Army, Department of the
Fifth Headquarters
Fort Sam Houston, Texas 78234

Army, Department of the
Washington, D.C. 20310

Army Training Support Center
Fort Eustis, Virginia 23604

Association-Sterling Films
(Addresses listed in local Telephone Directories)

Audiovisual Archives Division
National Archives and Records Service
Washington, D.C. 20408

Bierce Library
University of Akron
Buchtel Ave. and College St.
Akron, Ohio 44325

Bureau of Education for the Handicapped
Division of Media Services
Department of Health, Education, and Welfare
Washington, D.C. 20201

Bureau of Mines
  see: Mines, Bureau of
      Mining Safety and Health Administration

Bureau of Radiological Health
Food and Drug Administration
Public Health Service
Department of Health, Education, and Welfare
Rockville, Maryland 20852

Center for Disease Control
Public Health Service
Department of Health, Education, and Welfare
Atlanta, Georgia 30333

Civil Aeronautics Board
1825 Connecticut Avenue
Washington, D.C. 20428

Coast Guard
  see: U.S. Coast Guard

Commerce, Department of
Domestic and International Business Administration
Office of Energy Programs
Office of Field Operations
National Industrial Energy Council
Washington, D.C. 20230

Commerce, Department of
Washington, D.C. 20230

Community Services Administration
Washington, D.C. 20425

Consumer Affairs, Office of
Department of Health Education, and Welfare
Washington, D.C. 20201

Consumer Education and Awareness
Consumer Product Safety Commission
Washington, D.C. 20207

Consumer Inquiries
(HFG-20)
Food and Drug Administration
5600 Fishers Lane
Rockville, Maryland 20857

Consumer Product Safety Commission
Washington, D.C. 20207

Defense, Department of
Washington, D.C. 20301

Dental Training Center
Veterans Administration
Washington, D.C. 20420

Domestic and International Business Administration
  see: Commerce, Department of
      Domestic and International Business Administration

Drugs, Bureau of
Food and Drug Administration
Public Health Service
Washington, D.C. 20204

Drug Enforcement Administration
Department of Justice
Washington, D.C. 20230

Eastman Kodak
International Museum of Photography at George Eastman House
(Formerly George Eastman House Museum)
900 E. Avenue
Rochester, New York 14601

Energy, Department of (DOE)
Film Library
P.O. Box 62
Oak Ridge, Tennessee 37830

Energy, Department of (DOE)
Washington, D.C. 20585

Education for the Handicapped, Bureau of
Office of Education
Washington, D.C. 20201

Environmental Protection Agency
Office of Public Awareness (A-107)
Washington, D.C. 20460

Environmental Research Center
Environmental Protection Agency
Washington, D.C. 20460

Environmental Research Laboratories
Department of Commerce
Boulder, Colorado 80302

Federal Emergency Management Agency
Washington, D.C. 20472

Federal Aviation Administration
Department of Transportation
Washington, D.C. 20590

Federal Highway Administration
Washington, D.C. 20591

Federal Maritime Commission
Washington, D.C. 20573

Fish and Wildlife Service
  see: U.S. Fish and Wildlife Service

Food and Drug Administration
5600 Fishers Lane
Rockville, Maryland 20857

Fifth United States Army Headquarters
  see: Army, Department of

Food and Nutrition Information and Educational Materials Center
National Agricultural Library
Room 304
Beltsville, Maryland 20705

Food and Nutrition Service
Department of Agriculture
Washington, D.C. 20505

Food Safety and Quality Service
Department of Agriculture
Washington, D.C. 20505

Forest Service, Department of Agriculture
Washington, D.C. 20250

Forest Service, Eastern Region (Milwaukee, Wisconsin)
USDA c/o John Hall Films Service
Milwaukee, Wisconsin 53209

Film Service, Pacific Northwest Region (Portland, Oregon)
USDA—Forest Service Pacific Northwest Region's Information Office
P.O. Box 3623
Portland, Oregon 97208

Health and Human Services, Department of
Bethesda, Maryland 20209

Health Resources Administration
Public Health Service
Hyattsville, Maryland 20782

Health Services Administration
Department of Health, Education, and Welfare
Washington, D.C. 20201

Housing and Urban Development, Department of
Office of Public Affairs
Washington, D.C. 20410

Indian Affairs, Bureau of
Department of the Interior
Washington, D.C. 20240

Interdepartmental Committee on Visual and Auditory Materials for Distribution Abroad
U.S. International Communication Agency
Washington, D.C. 20547

Interior, Department of the
Washington, D.C. 20547

International Development Cooperation Agency, U.S.
Washington, D.C. 20522

Justice, Department of
Washington, D.C. 20530

International Cancer Research Data Bank (ICRDB)
Office of International Institute
Blair Building, Room 114
Bethesda, Maryland 20014

International Communication Agency, U.S.
United States of America
1776 Pennsylvania Avenue
Washington, D.C. 20547

Labor, Department of
Washington, D.C. 20210

Library of Congress
Division of the Blind and Physically Handicapped
Washington, D.C. 20540

Library of Congress
Motion Picture, Broadcasting and Recorded Sound Division
Washington, D.C. 20540

Law Enforcement Assistance Administration
Department of Justice
Washington, D.C. 20531

Medicine and Surgery, Veterans Administration
Washington, D.C. 20420

Military Academy
  see: U.S. Military Academy
    (West Point)

Mental Retardation, President's Committee on
U.S. Department of Health, Education, and Welfare
5400 Fishers Lane
Rockville, Maryland 20852

Mines, Bureau of
Department of the Interior
Washington, D.C. 20240

Mining Safety and Health Administration
Department of Labor
4800 Forbes Avenue
Pittsburgh, Pennsylvania 15213

Minnesota Department of Natural Resources
Bureau of Information and Education
350 Centennial Building
658 Cedar Street
St. Paul, Minnesota 55101

Modern Talking Service
(Addresses listed in local Telephone Directories)

Museum of History and Technology
  see: Smithsonian Institution

Museum of Natural History
  see: Smithsonian Institution

National Aeronautics and Space Administration (NASA)
Washington, D.C. 20546

National Aerospace Museum
  see: Smithsonian Institution

National Audiovisual Center
National Archives and Records Service
General Services Administration
Washington, D.C. 20409

National Bureau of Standards
Public Information Division
Department of Commerce
Washington, D.C. 20230

National Commission on Libraries and Information Science
1717 K Street, N.W., Suite 601
Washington, D.C. 20036

National Cancer Institute
National Institutes of Health
Bethesda, Maryland 20205

National Center on Child Abuse and Neglect
Administration of Children, Youth, and Families
Department of Health, Education, and Welfare
Washington, D.C. 20201

National Clearinghouse for Drug Abuse Information
Alcohol, Drug Abuse, and Mental Health Administration
Department of Health, Education, and Welfare
5400 Fishers Lane
Rockville, Maryland 20852

National Endowment of the Humanities
Room 830
806 15th Street, NW
Washington, D.C. 20506

National Foundation of the Arts and the Humanities
Washington, D.C. 20506

National Heart, Lung, and Blood Institute
National High Blood Pressure Educational Program
120/80 National Institutes of Health
Bethesda, Maryland 20205

National High Blood Pressure Education Program
 see: National Heart, Lung, and Blood Institute

National Highway and Safety Administration
Department of Transportation
Washington, D.C. 20590

National Institute for Occupational Safety and Health (NIOSH)
Taft Research Center
4767 Columbia Parkway
Cincinnati, Ohio 45226

National Institute of Arthritis, Metabolism, and Digestive Diseases
National Institutes of Health
Bethesda, Maryland 20205

National Institute of Child Health and Human Development
National Institutes of Health
Bethesda, Maryland 20205

National Institute of Education
Washington, D.C. 20208

National Institute of Environmental Health Sciences
Research Triangle Park, North Carolina 27709

National Institute of Mental Health
Alcohol, Drug Abuse, and Mental Health Administration
U.S. Department of Health Education, and Welfare
5400 Fishers Lane
Rockville, Maryland 20852

National Institute on Drug Abuse
Office of Communications and Public Affairs
U.S. Department of Health, Education, and Welfare
5400 Fishers Lane
Rockville, Maryland 20852

National Institute of Neurological and Communicative Disorders and Stroke
National Institutes of Health
Bethesda, Maryland 20205

National Institutes of Health
Bethesda, Maryland 20205

National Library of Medicine (NLM)
8600 Rockville Pike
Bethesda, Maryland 20205

National Medical Audiovisual Center (NMAC)
8600 Rockville Pike
Bethesda, Maryland 20205

National Oceanic and Atmospheric Administration
Department of Commerce
Rockville, Maryland 20205

The National Safety Council
245 N. Michigan Avenue
Chicago, Illinois 60611

National Science Foundation
Washington, D.C. 20550

National Technical Information Service (NTIS)
Department of Commerce
Springfield, Virginia 22161

Naval Health Sciences Education and Training Command
  see: Navy, Department of

Navy, Department of the
Naval Health Sciences Education and Training Command
Audiovisual Resources Section
National Naval Medical Center
Bethesda, Maryland 20014

Nuclear Regulatory Commission
Washington, D.C. 20555

Office of Consumer Affairs
  see: Consumer Affairs, Office of

Office of Education
Department of Health, Education, and Welfare
Washington, D.C. 20202

Office of Human Development
National Institute of Child Health and Human Development
National Institutes of Health
Bethesda, Maryland 20205

Office of Personnel Management
Office of Public Affairs
Washington, D.C. 20415

Physical Fitness and Sports, President's Council on
U.S. Department of Health, Education, and Welfare
5400 Fishers Lane
Rockville, Maryland 20852

President's Committee on Physical Fitness and Sports
  see: Physical Fitness and Sports

Prisons, Bureau of
Department of Justice
320 First Street, N.W.
Washington, D.C. 20530

Public Health Service
Department of Health, Education, and Welfare
200 Independence Avenue, S.W.
Washington, D.C. 20201

Rehabilitation Services Administration
Office of Human Development
U.S. Department of Health, Education, and Welfare
Washington, D.C. 20201

Smithsonian Institution
Office of Photographic Services/Museum of History and Technology/
  Aerospace/Natural History
Washington, D.C. 20560

Social Rehabilitation Service
Department of Health, Education, and Welfare
Washington, D.C. 20201

Superintendent of Documents
Government Printing Office
Washington, D.C. 20402

U.S. Coast Guard
Department of Transportation
Washington, D.C. 20590

U.S. Fish and Wildlife Service
Office of Public Affairs
Washington, D.C. 20240

U.S. Military Academy
West Point, New York 10996

Veterans Administration
  see also: Dental Training Center
          Veterans Administration

Veterans Administration
Medical Center
Medical Media Division—Central Office
Washington, D.C. 20420

Veterans Administration
Washington, D.C. 20420

West Point Academy
  see: U.S. Military Academy

Indexes

Title Index

Adult Group Leader Guide for Use with DIAL A-L-C-O-H-O-L and Jackson Junior High: Two Film Series on Alcohol Education
AoA Catalog of Films on Aging
AoA Fact Sheet: Audiovisual Materials Sponsored by the Administration on Aging
Army Films for Non-Profit Use
Audio-Visual Materials Catalog—Arthritis Information Clearinghouse
Audiovisual Aids Directory of the Rehabilitation Research and Training Centers: Audiotape, Film, Slides, Videotape
Audiovisual Aids for High Blood Pressure Education
Audiovisual Catalog—NIDA Resource Center
Audiovisual Catalog of the National Highway Traffic Safety Administration
Audiovisual Guide to the Catalog of the Food and Nutrition Information and Educational Materials Center
Audiovisual Materials in Dental Auxiliary Education

Bimonthly List of Publications and Audiovisuals
Braille Book Review

Cancer Guide
Career Education: Selected U.S. Government Audiovisuals
Cassette Books
Catalog of Audio-Visual Aids in Hypertension
Catalog of Educational Captioned Films for the Deaf
Catalog of Family Planning Materials
Catalog of Films Available from Agencies: The U.S. Department of Commerce Serving the Nation
Catalog of the FDA Publications and Audiovisual Materials for Consumers
Catalog of the United States Coast Guard Films
Catalog of Training Films and Other Media for Special Education
Child Abuse and Neglect Audiovisual Materials
Criminal Justice Audiovisual Materials Directory

Dental Training Films
Dentistry: A Select List of the U.S. Government Audiovisual Materials

Title Index

Directory of Cancer Research Information Resources
Directory of U.S. Government Audiovisual Personnel
Disaster Preparedness: Publications, Films, and Other Audio-Visual Materials from the National Weather Service
Documentary Film Classics Produced by the United States Government
Drug Abuse Films
Drug Abuse Prevention Films: A Multicultural Film Catalog

Educational Media Resources on Egypt
Energy Efficiency Sharing: Business-to-Business Program to Facilitate Exchange of Energy Management Technology and Techniques
Energy Films Catalog
Engineering: Selected U.S. Government Audiovisuals
Environmental Movies and Slides from EPA

FAA Film Catalog [for Public Use]
Federal Emergency Management Agency Motion Picture Catalog
Film Archives on Child Development—The Inauguration of the Child Development Archives
Film Catalog
Film Catalog 1980. Pacific Northern Region
Film Fare: A Catalog of Films and Filmstrips Produced by the U.S. Department of Housing and Urban Development
Film Guide to Reproduction and Development: A Guide to Selected Films on Reproductive and Developmental Biology for Graduate and Undergraduate Programs in the Biomedical Sciences
Film Resources on Japan
Films: Free from the National Bureau of Standards
Forest Service Films Available on Loan to the Public for Educational Purposes

Guide to Audio-Visual Aids for Courses in the History of Latin American Civilization in Higher Education Institutions, A
Guide to Audiovisual Aids for Spanish-Speaking Americans

Health, 1980-81
Health: A Selected List of Books that Have Appeared in Talking Book Topics and Braille Book Review

In Focus: Alcohol and Alcoholism Media
Index to Army Motion Pictures for Public Non-Profit Use
Indians in the United States: Select Audiovisual Records

Library of Congress Catalogs: Audiovisual Materials
Libros Parlantes (Talking Book Topics)
List of Audiovisual Materials Produced by the United States Government for Business and Government Management, A
List of Audiovisual Materials Produced by the United States Government for Consumer Education, A
List of Audiovisual Materials Produced by the United States Government for Drug Abuse Prevention, A
List of Audiovisual Materials Produced by the United States Government for Emergency Medical Service, A
List of Audiovisual Materials Produced by the United States Government for Environment and Energy Conservation, A

List of Audiovisual Materials Produced by the United States Government for Fire/Law Enforcement, A
List of Audiovisual Materials Produced by the United States Government for Flight and Meteorology, A
List of Audiovisual Materials Produced by the United States Government for Foreign Language Instruction, A
List of Audiovisual Materials Produced by the United States Government for Industrial Safety, A
List of Audiovisual Materials Produced by the United States Government for Nursing, A
List of Audiovisual Materials Produced by the United States Government for Social Issues, A
List of Audiovisual Materials Produced by the United States Government for Special Education, A
List of Audiovisual Materials Produced by the United States Government in History, A
List of Audiovisual Materials Produced by the United States Government—Spanish Language Soundtracks, A
List of Educational Aids
Listing of Educational Materials for Use by Schools

Materials from the National Arts and the Handicapped Information Service: Annotated Bibliography
Media Resources Catalog
Medical Catalog of Selected Audiovisual Materials Produced by the United States Government
Medical Cinematography
Medical Film Catalog
Mental Retardation Film List
Motion Pictures, Films, and Audiovisual Information: Subject Bibliography

NASA Film List
National Library of Medicine Audiovisuals Catalog
National Library of Medicine AVLINE Catalog, 1975-1976
National Medical Audiovisual Center Catalog: Films for the Health Sciences
Natural Resources Department Films
Neurological and Sensory Disease Film Guide
1970 Film Reference Guide for Medicine and Allied Health Sciences
1969 Film Reference Guide for Medicine and Allied Sciences
1967 Public Health Service Film Catalog
NIOSH—Films and Filmstrips on Occupational Safety and Health
NMAC News: Selected Biomedical Audiovisuals
NOAA Motion Picture Films

Problems in Bibliographic Access to Non-Print Materials, Project Media Base: Final Report
Publications, Radio, Films, Slides, Fact Sheets, T.V.

Quarterly Update: A Comprehensive Listing of New Audiovisual Materials and Services Offered by the National Audiovisual Center

Radiological Health Training Resources Catalog
Recent Film Releases of the U.S. Department of Agriculture
Reference List of Audiovisual Materials Produced by the United States Government, A
Resource File: Practical Publications for Energy Management. A Reference Guide to Handbooks, Curricula, and Audiovisual Materials, The
Resources in Women's Educational Equity Non-Print Media and Materials

Title Index

Selected Audiovisuals on Mental Health
Selected Educational Media
Selected Films: Heart Disease, Cancer, and Stroke
Selected Guide to Audio-Visual Materials on Alcohol and Alcoholism, A
Selected List: Alcohol and Drug Problems
Smithsonian Slide Series. Slides. Filmstrips. Audiocassettes.
Source Book of Educational Materials for Radiation Therapy
Space Benefits: NASA Films and Publications Describing Benefits of Space and Technology
Special Education: Selected U.S. Audiovisuals

Talking Book Topics
35 Energy Films
Training Films [Mine Safety and Health Administration]

Union List of Audiovisuals in the Library Network of the Veterans Administration
United States Government Motion Pictures for Television Programs Submitted in 1980 and 1981 to *International Film and Television Events*

VA Film Catalog
Venereal Disease Films [For the General Public]
Video Tape Catalog Continuing Medical Education and Instruction (AHSUSA)
Viking Film Announcement

Where the Drug Films Are: A Guide to Evaluation Services and Distributors

Subject Index

ABUSE
Child
Police
Spouse
Women

    Child Abuse and Neglect Audiovisual Materials
    Film Archives on Child Development—The Inauguration of the Child Development Archives
    Criminal Justice Audiovisual Materials Directory
    Health
    Library of Congress Catalogs: Audiovisual Materials
    List of Audiovisual Materials Produced by the U.S. Government in History, A
    Media Resources Catalog
    National Library of Medicine Audiovisuals Catalog
    National Library of Medicine AVLINE Catalog
    National Medical Audiovisual Center Catalog: Films for the Health Sciences
    Resources in Women's Educational Equity Non-Profit Media and Materials
    Union List of Audiovisuals in the Library Network of the Veterans Administration

ACCIDENTS AND ACCIDENT PREVENTION

    Army Films for Non-Profit Use
    Audiovisual Catalog of National Highway Traffic Safety Administration
    Child Abuse and Neglect Audiovisual Materials
    Criminal Justice Audiovisual Materials Directory
    FAA Film Catalog
    Guide to Audiovisual Aids for Spanish-Speaking Americans
    Library of Congress Catalogs: Audiovisual Materials
    List of Audiovisual Materials Produced by the U.S. Government for Consumer Education, A
    List of Audiovisual Materials Produced by the U.S. Government for Flight and Meteorology, A
    Listing of Educational Materials for Use by Schools

Subject Index

ACCIDENTS AND ACCIDENT PREVENTION (continued)

    Medical Catalog of Selected Audiovisual Materials Produced by the U.S. Government
    National Library of Medicine Audiovisuals Catalog
    National Library of Medicine AVLINE Catalog
    National Medical Audiovisual Center Catalog: Films for the Health Sciences
    1970 Film Reference Guide for Medicine and Allied Health Sciences
    1969 Film Reference Guide for Medicine and Allied Sciences
    1967 Public Health Service Film Catalog
    Training Films [Mine Safety and Health Administration]
    Union List of Audiovisuals in the Library Network of the Veterans Administration
    VA Film Catalog

ACCLIMATIZATION
see CLIMATE

ACUPUNCTURE

In Focus: Alcohol and Alcoholism Media

AGED, AGING
see GERIATRICS

AGRICULTURE
Plants

    Audiovisual Guide to the Catalog of the Food and Nutrition Information and Educational Materials Center
    Bimonthly List of Publications and Audiovisuals
    Educational Media Resources in Egypt
    Energy Films Catalog
    Film Catalog 1980, Pacific Region
    Forest Service Films Available on Loan to the Public for Educational Purposes
    Guide to Audio-Visual Aids for Courses in the History of Latin American Civilization in Higher Education Institutions, A
    Library of Congress Catalogs: Audiovisual Materials
    List of Audiovisual Materials Produced by the U.S. Government for Industrial Safety, A
    Medical Catalog of Selected Audiovisual Materials Produced by the U.S. Government
    NASA Film List
    Natural Resources Department Films
    1970 Film Reference Guide for Medicine and Allied Health Sciences
    1969 Film Reference Guide for Medicine and Allied Sciences
    1967 Public Health Service Film Catalog
    Quarterly Update: A Comprehensive Listing of New Audiovisual Materials and Services Offered by the National Audiovisual Center
    Recent Film Releases of the U.S. Department of Agriculture
    Reference List of Audiovisual Materials Produced by the U.S. Government, A

ALCOHOL
see DRUG ABUSE

ANATOMY, HISTOLOGY, PHYSIOLOGY

Audiovisual Aids Directory of the Rehabilitation Research and Training Centers
Audiovisual Guide to the Catalog of the Food and Nutrition Information and Educational Materials Center
Audiovisual Materials in Dental Auxiliary Education
Dental Training Films
Dentistry: A Select List of U.S. Government Produced Audiovisual Materials
Film Catalog
In Focus: Alcohol and Alcoholism Media
Medical Film Catalog
National Library of Medicine Audiovisuals Catalog
National Library of Medicine AVLINE Catalog
National Medical Audiovisual Center Catalog: Films for the Health Sciences
Source of Educational Materials for Radiation Therapy
Union List of Audiovisuals in the Library Network of the Veterans Administration
VA Film Catalog

ANESTHESIOLOGY

Audiovisual Materials in Dental Auxiliary Education
Dentistry: A Select List of U.S. Government Produced Audiovisual Materials
Library of Congress Catalogs: Audiovisual Materials
Medical Film Catalog
National Library of Medicine AVLINE Catalog
National Medical Audiovisual Center Catalog: Films for the Health Sciences
Union List of Audiovisuals in the Library Network of the Veterans Administration

ANTHROPOLOGY AND ARCHEOLOGY

Educational Media Resources in Egypt
Film Resources in Japan
Guide to Audio-Visual Aids for Courses in the History of Latin American Civilization in Higher Education Institutions, A
Indians in the United States: Select Audiovisual Records
NASA Film List
Reference List of Audiovisual Materials Produced by the United States Government—Suppl., A
Smithsonian Slide Series. Slides. Filmstrips. Audiocassettes. Booklets.

ARCHEOLOGY
see ANTHROPOLOGY...

ARTHRITIS

Audiovisual Aids Directory of the Rehabilitation Research and Training
Audio Visual Materials Catalog—Arthritis Information Clearinghouse
Health: A Selected List of Books that Have Appeared in Braille Book Review, and Talking Book Topics
Library of Congress Catalogs: Audiovisual Materials
National Library of Medicine Audiovisuals Catalog
National Library of Medicine AVLINE Catalog
Reference List of Audiovisual Materials Produced by the U.S. Government, A

Subject Index

ARTHRITIS (continued)

    Union List of Audiovisual Materials in the Library Network of the Veterans Administration, A

ATMOSPHERE
    see CLIMATE...

ATOMIC ENERGY
    see also ENERGY

    Energy Films Catalog
    Engineering: Selected U.S. Government Audiovisuals
    Film Resources on Japan
    Medical Catalog of Selected Audiovisual Materials Produced by the U.S. Government
    Reference List of Audiovisual Materials Produced by the U.S. Government, A

AUDIOLOGY
    see also OTORHINOLARYNGOLOGY

    Catalog of Training Films and Other Media for Special Education

AVIATION AND AVIATION MEDICINE

    Audiovisual Catalog of National Highway Traffic Safety Administration
    FAA Film Catalog
    Federal Emergency Management Agency Motion Picture Catalog
    In Focus: Alcohol and Alcoholism Media
    Index of Army Motion Pictures for Public Non-Profit Use
    List of Audiovisual Materials Produced by the U.S. Government for Flight and Meteorology, A
    Medical Catalog of Selected Audiovisual Materials Produced by the United States Government
    Medical Film Catalog
    NASA Film List
    1970 Film Reference Guide for Medicine and Allied Health Sciences
    Reference List of Audiovisual Materials Produced by the U.S. Government, A
    Smithsonian Slide Series: Slides. Filmstrips. Audiocassettes. Booklets.

AVIATION MEDICINE
    see AVIATION...

BEHAVIOR MODIFICATION
    see MENTAL HEALTH

BIBLIOGRAPHY (Nondescriptive—Print and Nonprint)

    Adult Group Leader Guide for Use with Dial A-L-C-O-H-O-L and Jackson Junior High
    AoA Fact Sheet: Audiovisual Materials Sponsored by the Administration on Aging
    Audio-Visual Materials Catalog—Arthritis Information Clearinghouse
    Directory of Cancer Research Information Resources
    Documentary Film Classics Produced by the United States Government

BIBLIOGRAPHY ... (continued)

Energy Efficiency Sharing: Business-To-Business Program to Facilitate Exchange of Energy Management Technology and Techniques
Film Archives on Child Development—The Inauguration of the Child Development Archives
Guide to Audio-Visual Aids for Courses in the History of Latin American Civilization in Higher Education Institutions, A
Materials from the National Arts and the Handicapped Information
Medical Cinematography
Motion Pictures, Films, and Audiovisual Information: Subject Bibliography
Quarterly Update: A Comprehensive Listing of New Audiovisual Materials and Service Offered by the National Audiovisual Center
Resource File: Practical Publications for Energy Management. A Reference Guide to Handbooks, Curricula, and Audiovisual Materials, The
Resources in Women's Educational Equity Non-Print Media and Materials
Smithsonian Slide Series. Slides. Filmstrips. Audiocassettes. Booklets.
Source Book of Educational Materials for Radiation Therapy
United States Government Motion Pictures and Television Programs Submitted in 1980 and 1981 to International Film and Television Events

BIOLOGY

Army Films for Non-Profit Use
Catalog of Films Available from Agencies: The U.S. Department of Commerce
Energy Films Catalog
Film Guide on Reproduction and Development
Library of Congress Catalogs: Audiovisual Materials
Medical Catalog of Selected Audiovisual Materials Produced by the U.S. Government
National Library of Medicine Audiovisual Catalog
National Library of Medicine AVLINE Catalog
National Medical Audiovisual Center Catalog: Films for the Health Sciences
1970 Film Reference Guide fo Medicine and Allied Health Sciences
1969 Film Reference Guide for Medicine and Allied Sciences
1967 Public Health Service Film Catalog
Reference List of Audiovisual Materials Produced by the U.S. Government, A
Resources in Women's Educational Equity Non-Print Media and Materials
Selected Audiovisuals on Mental Health
Selected Educational Media
Selected Guide to Audio-Visual Materials on Alcohol and Alcoholism, A
Selected List: Alcohol and Drug Problems
Source of Educational Materials for Radiation Therapy
Union List of Audiovisuals in the Library Network of the Veterans Administration

BIRTH CONTROL
see FAMILY PLANNING

BIRTH DEFECTS
see GENETICS

Subject Index

BLOOD

Army Films for Non-Profit Use
Audiovisual Aids Directory of the Rehabilitation Research and Training Centers
Index to Army Motion Pictures for Public Non-Profit Use
Library of Congress Catalogs: Audiovisual Materials
List of Audiovisual Materials Produced by the U.S. Government for Flight and Meteorology, A
List of Educational Aids
National Library of Medicine Audiovisuals Catalog
National Medical Audiovisual Center Catalog: Films for the Health Sciences
National Library of Medicine AVLINE Catalog
Source Book of Educational Materials for Radiation Therapy
Union List of Audiovisuals in the Library Network of the Veterans Administration

BLOOD PRESSURE
see HYPERTENSION

BUSINESS AND ECONOMICS
see ORGANIZATION AND ADMINISTRATION

CANCER
see NEOPLASMS

CARDIOVASCULAR SYSTEM

Audiovisual Aids Directory of the Rehabilitation Research and Training Centers
Guide to Audiovisual Aids for Spanish-Speaking Americans
Health: A Selected List of Books that Have Appeared in Braille Book Review, and Talking Book Topics
Index to Army Motion Pictures for Public Non-Profit Use
List of Audiovisual Materials Produced by the U.S. Government for Emergency Medical Services, A
List of Educational Aids
Library of Congress Catalogs: Audiovisual Materials
National Library of Medicine Audiovisuals Catalog
National Library of Medicine AVLINE Catalog
National Medical Audiovisual Center Catalog: Films for the Health Sciences
1970 Film Reference Guide for Medicine and Allied Health Sciences
1969 Film Reference Guide for Medicine and Allied Sciences
1967 Public Health Service Film Catalog
Source Book of Educational Materials for Radiation Therapy
Training Films [Mine Safety and Health Administration]
Union List of Audiovisuals in the Library Network of the Veterans Administration
VA Film Catalog
Video Tape Catalog Continuing Medical Education and Instruction (AHSUSA)

CAREERS
Vocational Training

Audiovisual Guide to the Catalog of the Food and Nutrition Information and Educational Materials Center
Career Education: Selected U.S. Government Audiovisuals

Subject Index

CAREERS (continued)

    Catalog of Educational Captioned Films for the Deaf
    Energy Films Catalog
    Medical Catalog of Selected Audiovisual Materials Produced by the U.S. Government
    Quarterly Update: A Comprehensive Listing of New Audiovisual Materials and Services Offered by the National Audiovisual Center
    Reference List of Audiovisual Materials Produced by the United States Government—Suppl., A
    Union List of Audiovisuals in the Library Network of the Veterans Administration
    VA Film Catalog

CASE REPORT

    Audio Visual Materials Catalog—Arthritis Information Clearinghouse
    Audiovisual Catalog of National Highway Traffic Safety Administration
    Criminal Justice Audiovisual Materials Directory
    Directory of Cancer Research Information Resources
    Health: A Selected List of Books that Have Appeared in Braille Book Review, and Talking Book Topics
    In Focus: Alcohol and Alcoholism Media
    Index to Army Motion Pictures for Public Non Profit Use
    Radiological Health Training Resources Catalog

CEREBRAL PALSY
  see **HANDICAPPED**
      NEUROLOGY

CHEMICAL WARFARE
  see **CHEMICAL, BIOLOGICAL...(Miscellaneous)**

CHEMISTRY AND CHEMICALS
  see also **POISONING**
      TOXICOLOGY

    Army Films for Non-Profit Use
    Catalog of Films Available from Agencies: The U.S. Department of Commerce Serving the Nation
    Films: Free from the National Bureau of Standards
    Library of Congress Catalogs: Audiovisual Materials
    List of Audiovisual Materials Produced by the U.S. Government for Flight and Meteorology, A
    List of Educational Aids
    Medical Catalog of Selected Audiovisual Materials Produced by the U.S. Government
    National Library of Medicine Audiovisuals Catalog
    National Library of Medicine AVLINE Catalog
    National Medical Audiovisual Center Catalog: Films for the Health Sciences
    NIOSH—Films and Filmstrips on Occupational Safety and Health
    1970 Film Reference Guide for Medicine and Allied Health Sciences
    1969 Film Reference Guide for Medicine and Allied Sciences
    1967 Public Health Service Films Catalog
    Publications, Radio, Films, Slides, Fact Sheets, T.V.
    Reference List of Audiovisual Materials Produced by the U.S. Government, A

CHEMISTRY AND CHEMICALS (continued)

    Selected Audiovisuals on Mental Health
    Selected Guide to Audio-Visual Materials on Alcohol and Alcoholism, A
    Source Book of Educational Materials for Radiation Therapy
    Union List of Audiovisuals in the Library Network of the Veterans Administration

CLERGY
  see RELIGION

CLIMATE, ACCLIMATIZATION, ATMOSPHERE, METEOROLOGY, WEATHER

    Army Films for Non-Profit Use
    Bimonthly List of Publications and Audiovisuals
    Career Education: Selected U.S. Government Audiovisuals
    Disaster Preparedness: Publications, Films and Other Audio-Visual Materials from the Weather Service
    Educational Media Resources in Egypt
    FAA Film Catalog
    Film Catalog 1980. Pacific Northern Region
    Film Resources on Japan
    List of Audiovisual Materials Produced by the U.S. Government for Flight and Meteorology, A
    Medical Film Catalog
    NASA Film List
    NOAA Motion Picture Films
    Quarterly Update: A Comprehensive Listing of Audiovisual Materials and Services Offered by the National Audiovisual Center (NAC)
    Recent Film Releases of the U.S. Department of Agriculture
    Resource File: Practical Publications for Energy Management. A Reference Guide to Handbooks, Curricula, and Audiovisual Materials, The

COMMUNICABLE DISEASES

    AoA Catalog of Films on Aging
    Catalog of Family Planning Materials
    Guide to Audiovisual Aids for Spanish-Speaking Americans
    Health: A Selected List of Books that Have Appeared in Braille Book Review, and Talking Book Topics
    Library of Congress Catalogs: Audiovisual Materials
    List of Educational Aids
    National Library of Medicine Audiovisuals Catalog
    National Library of Medicine AVLINE Catalog
    National Medical Audiovisual Center Catalog: Films for the Health Sciences
    Recent Film Releases of the U.S. Department of Agriculture
    Source Book of Educational Materials for Radiation Therapy
    Union List of Audiovisuals in the Library Network of the Veterans Administration
    VA Film Catalog
    Venereal Disease Films for the General Public

COMMUNITY HEALTH
see also ABUSE
CRISIS INTERVENTION
DRUG ABUSE
EMERGENCIES
GOVERNMENT PROGRAMS
PUBLIC HEALTH

AoA Catalog of Films on Aging
Adult Group Leader Guide for the Use with DIAL A-L-C-O-H-O-L and Junior High
Audiovisual Aids Directory of the Rehabilitation Research and Training Centers
Audiovisual Catalog—NIDA Resource Center
Audiovisual Guide to the Catalog of the Food and Nutrition Information and Educational Materials Center
Audiovisual Materials in Dental Auxiliary Education
Catalog of Family Planning Materials
Catalog of the FDA Publications and Audiovisual Materials for Consumers
Catalog of Training Films and Other Media for Special Education
Child Abuse and Neglect Audiovisual Materials
Criminal Justice Audiovisual Materials Directory
Directory of Cancer Research Information Resources
Documentary Film Classics Produced by the U.S. Government
Drug Abuse Films
Drug Abuse Prevention Films: A Multicultural Film Catalog
Guide to Audiovisual Aids for Spanish-Speaking Americans
In Focus: Alcohol and Alcoholism Media
List of Audiovisual Materials Produced by the U.S. Government for Business and Government Management, A
List of Audiovisual Materials Produced by the U.S. Government for Emergency Medical Service, A
Media Resources Catalog
National Library of Medicine Audiovisuals Catalog
National Medical Audiovisual Center Catalog: Films for the Health Sciences
Reference List of Audiovisual Materials Produced by the U.S. Government, A
Resource File: Practical Publications for Energy Management. A Reference Guide to Handbooks, Curricula, and Audiovisual Materials, The
Selected Audiovisuals on Mental Health
Selected Guide to Audio-Visual Materials on Alcohol and Alcoholism, A
Special Education: Selected U.S. Government Audiovisuals
Venereal Disease Films for the General Public

COMPUTERS
see TECHNOLOGY

CONSERVATION OF NATURAL RESOURCES
see ENERGY

CONSUMER
see also GOVERNMENT PROGRAMS

Catalog of Educational Captioned Films for the Deaf
Catalog of the FDA Publications and Audiovisual Materials for Consumers

Subject Index

CONSUMER (continued)

    Energy Films Catalog
    Films: Free from the National Bureau of Standards
    List of Audiovisual Materials Produced by the U.S. Government for Business and Government Management, A
    List of Audiovisual Materials Produced by the U.S. Government for Consumer Education, A
    Listing of Educational Materials for Use by Schools
    Publications, Radio, Films, Slides, Fact Sheets, T.V.
    Quarterly Update: A Comprehensive Listing of New Audiovisual Materials and Services Offered by the National Audiovisual Center
    Radiological Health Training Resources Catalog
    Resource File: Practical Publications for Energy Management. A Reference Guide to Handbooks, Curricula, and Audiovisual Materials, The
    Selected List: Alcohol and Drug Problems
    Source Book of Educational Materials for Radiation Therapy

CONTRACEPTIVES
    see **FAMILY PLANNING**

COSMETICS
    see **CONSUMER**

COUNSELING

    Adult Group Leader Guide for the Use with DIAL A-L-C-O-H-O-L and Jackson Junior High
    Audiovisual Aids Directory of the Rehabilitation Research and Training Centers
    Audiovisual Catalog—NIDA Resource Center
    Catalog of Educational Captioned Films for the Deaf
    Child Abuse and Neglect Audiovisual Materials
    Drug Abuse Films
    Drug Abuse Prevention Films: A Multicultural Film Catalog
    In Focus: Alcohol and Alcoholism Media
    List of Audiovisual Materials Produced by the U.S. Government for Drug Abuse Prevention, A
    List of Audiovisual Materials Produced by the U.S. Government for Special Education, A
    Media Resources Catalog
    Resources in Women's Educational Equity Non-Print Media and Materials
    Source Book of Educational Materials for Radiation Therapy
    Special Education: Selected U.S. Government Audiovisuals
    Union List of Audiovisuals in the Library Network of the Veterans Administration

CRIMINAL LAW
    see **JURISPRUDENCE**

CRISIS INTERVENTION
    see also **EMERGENCIES**

    Adult Group Leader Guide for the Use with DIAL A-L-C-O-H-O-L and Jackson Junior High

CRISIS INTERVENTION (continued)

    Audiovisual Catalog—NIDA Resource Center
    Bimonthly List of Publications and Audiovisuals
    Catalog of Family Planning Materials
    Child Abuse and Neglect Audiovisual Materials
    Drug Abuse Prevention Films: A Multicultural Film Catalog
    FAA Film Catalog for Public Use
    In Focus: Alcohol and Alcoholism Media
    Index of Army Motion Pictures for Public Non-Profit Use
    Library of Congress Catalogs: Audiovisual Materials
    Listing of Educational Materials for Use by Schools
    1967 Public Health Service Film Catalog
    Quarterly Update: A Comprehensive Listing of New Audiovisual Materials and Services Offered by the National Audiovisual Center
    Resources in Women's Educational Equity Non-Print Media and Materials
    Selected Audiovisuals on Mental Health
    Veneral Disease Films for the General Public

CHROMATOGRAPHY

    Source Book of Educational Materials for Radiation Therapy

CRIME
    see CRIMES... (Miscellaneous)

CYTOLOGY AND TISSUE CULTURE

    National Library of Medicine Audiovisuals Catalog
    National Library of Medicine AVLINE Catalog
    National Medical Audiovisual Center Catalog: Films for the Health Sciences
    Union List of Audiovisuals in the Library Network of the Veterans Administration

DEATH
    see also THANATOLOGY

DENTISTRY

    Army Films for Non-Profit Use
    Audiovisual Guide to the Catalog of the Food and Nutrition Information and Educational Materials Center
    Audiovisual Materials in Dental Auxiliary Education
    Dental Training Films
    Dentistry: A Select List of U.S. Government Produced Audiovisual Materials
    Directory of Cancer Research Information Programs
    Films: Free from the National Bureau of Standards
    Guide to Audiovisual Aids for Spanish-Speaking Americans
    Index of Army Motion Pictures for Public Non-profit Use
    List of Audiovisual Materials Produced by the U.S. Government for Business and Government Personnel, A
    List of Audiovisual Materials Produced by the U.S. Government for Consumer Education, A
    List of Educational Aids

Subject Index

DENTISTRY (continued)

    Medical Catalog of Selected Audiovisual Materials Produced by the U.S. Government
    National Library of Medicine Audiovisuals Catalog
    National Library of Medicine AVLINE Catalog
    National Medical Audiovisual Center Catalog: Films for the Health Sciences
    1967 Public Health Service Film Catalog
    Quarterly Update: A Comprehensive Listing of New Audiovisual Materials and Services Offered by the National Audiovisual Center (NAC)
    Reference List of Audiovisual Materials Produced by the U.S. Government, A
    Reference List of Audiovisual Materials Produced by the U.S. Government—Suppl., A
    Union List of Audiovisuals in the Library Network of the Veterans Administration
    VA Film Catalog
    Video Tape Catalog Continuing Medical Education and Instruction (AHSUSA)

DERMATOLOGY
    Skin

    Army Films for Non-Profit Use
    Index of Army Motion Pictures for Public Non-Profit Use
    Library of Congress Catalogs: Audiovisual Materials
    List of Audiovisual Materials Produced by the U.S. Government for Business and Government Management, A
    List of Educational Aids
    Medical Film Catalog
    National Library of Medicine AVLINE Catalog
    NIOSH—Films and Filmstrips on Occupational Safety and Health
    Union List of Audiovisuals in the Library Network of the Veterans Administration
    Video Tape Catalog Continuing Medical Education and Instruction (AHSUSA)

DIET
    see NUTRITION...

DIGESTIVE SYSTEM

    National Library of Medicine Audiovisuals Catalog
    National Library of Medicine AVLINE Catalog
    National Medical Audiovisuals Center Catalog: Films for the Health Sciences
    1970 Film Reference Guide for Medicine and Allied Health Sciences
    1967 Public Health Service Film Catalog
    Union List of Audiovisuals in the Library Network of the Veterans Administration

DISASTERS
    Natural
    War

    Army Films for Non-Profit Use
    Catalog of Educational Captioned Films for the Deaf
    Catalog of Films Available from Agencies: The U.S. Department of Commerce Serving the Nation
    Catalog of the United States Coast Guard Films

Subject Index

DISASTERS (continued)

    Disaster Preparedness: Publications, Films and Other Audiovisual Materials from the Weather Service
    Educational Media Resources in Egypt
    Federal Emergency Management Agency Motion Picture Catalog
    Forest Service Films Available on Loan to the Public for Educational Purposes
    Indians in the United States: Select Audiovisual Records
    List of Audiovisual Materials Produced by the U.S. Government in History, A
    List of Audiovisual Materials Produced by the U.S. Government for Emergency Service, A
    List of Audiovisual Materials Produced by the U.S. Government for Fire/Law Enforcement, A
    List of Audiovisual Materials Produced by the U.S. Government for Flight and Meteorology, A
    List of Educational Aids
    NASA Film List
    National Library of Medicine AVLINE Catalog
    Natural Resources Department Films
    1969 Film Reference Guide for Medicine and Allied Sciences
    1967 Public Health Service Film Catalog
    NOAA Motion Picture Films
    Recent Film Releases of the U.S. Department of Agriculture
    Selected Educational Media
    Space Benefits: NASA Films and Publications Describing Benefits of Space Technology

DOWN'S SYNDROME
see also **HANDICAPPED**
    MENTAL HEALTH
    MENTAL RETARDATION

    Audiovisual Aids Directory of the Rehabilitation Research and Training Centers

DRUG ABUSE
    Alcohol
    Drugs
    Smoking
    Tobacco

    Adult Group Leader Guide for the Use with DIAL A-L-C-O-H-O-L and Jackson Junior High
    Audiovisuals Aids Directory of the Rehabilitation Research and Training Centers
    Audiovisual Catalog—NIDA Resource Center
    Audiovisual Catalog of the National Highway Traffic Safety Administration
    Audiovisual Guide to the Catalog of the Food and Nutrition Information and Educational Materials Center
    Cancer Film Guide
    Catalog of the FDA Publications and Audiovisual Materials for Consumers
    Child Abuse and Neglect Audiovisual Materials
    Criminal Justice Audiovisual Materials Directory
    Drug Abuse Films
    Drug Abuse Prevention Films: A Multicultural Film Catalog

Subject Index

DRUG ABUSE (continued)

Guide to Audiovisual Aids for Spanish-Speaking Americans
Health
Health: A Selected List of Books that Have Appeared in Braille Book Review and Talking Book Topics
In Focus: Alcohol and Alcoholism Media
Index to Army motion Pictures for Public Non-Profit Use
Library of Congress Catalogs: Audiovisual Materials
List of Audiovisual Materials Produced by the U.S. Government for Consumer Education, A
List of Audiovisual Materials Produced by the U.S. Government for Drug Abuse Prevention, A
List of Audiovisual Materials Produced by the U.S. Government for Flight and Meteorology, A
List of Audiovisual Materials Produced by the U.S. Government—Spanish Language Soundtracks, A
Media Resources Catalog
Medical Catalog of Selected Audiovisual Materials Produced by the U.S. Government
Medical Film Catalog
National Library of Medicine Audiovisuals Catalog
National Library of Medicine AVLINE Catalog
National Medical Audiovisual Center Catalog: Films for the Health Sciences
Neurological and Sensory Disease Film Guide
1970 Film Reference Guide for Medicine and Allied Health Sciences
1969 Film Reference Guide for Medicine and Allied Sciences
1967 Public Health Service Film Catalog
Quarterly Update: A Comprehensive Listing of New Audiovisual Materials and Services Offered by the National Audiovisuals Center
Reference List to Audiovisual Materials Produced by the U.S. Government, A
Resources in Women's Educational Equity Non-Print Media and Materials
Selected Audiovisuals on Mental Health
Selected Films: Heart Disease, Cancer, and Stroke
Selected Guide to Audio-Visual Materials on Alcohol Issues, A
Selected List: Alcohol and Drug Problems
Union List of Audiovisuals in the Library Network of the Veterans Administration
VA Film Catalog
Video Tape Catalog Continuing Medical Education and Instruction (AHSUSA)
Where the Drug Films Are: A Guide to Evaluation Services and Distributors

DRUGS, PRESCRIPTION, NON-PRESCRIPTION (OTC)

Audio Visual Materials Catalog—Arthritis Information Clearinghouse
Audiovisual Aids Directory of the Rehabilitation Research and Training Centers
Audiovisual Aids for High Blood Pressure Education
Audiovisual Catalog of the National Highway Traffic Safety Administration
Audiovisual Guide to the Catalog of the Food and Nutrition Information and Educational Materials Center
Cancer Film Guide
Catalog of Audio-Visual Aids in Hypertension
Catalog of Family Planning Materials
Catalog of the FDA Publications and Audiovisual Materials for Consumers
Dental Training Films

DRUGS, PRESCRIPTION, NON-PRESCRIPTION (OTC) (continued)

    Dentistry: A Select List of U.S. Government Produced Audiovisual Materials
    Drug Abuse Films
    Guide to Audiovisual Aids for Spanish-Speaking Americans
    In Focus: Alcohol and Alcoholism Media
    Health
    Health: A Selected List of Books that Have Appeared in Braille Book Review, and Talking Book Topics
    Index of Army Motion Pictures for Public Non-Profit Use
    Library of Congress Catalogs: Audiovisual Materials
    List of Audiovisual Materials Produced by the U.S. Government for Nursing, A
    List of Educational Aids
    Medical Catalog of Selected Audiovisual Materials Produced by the U.S. Government
    Medical Film Catalog
    Mental Retardation Film List
    National Medical Audiovisual Center Catalog: Films for the Health Sciences
    National Library of Medicine Audiovisuals Catalog
    National Library of Medicine AVLINE Catalog
    Neurological and Sensory Disease Film Guide
    1970 Film Reference Guide for Medicine and Allied Health Sciences
    1969 Film Reference Guide for Medicine and Allied Sciences
    1967 Public Health Service Film Catalog
    Publications, Radio, Films, Slides, Fact Sheets, T.V.
    Quarterly Update: A Comprehensive Listing of New Audiovisual Materials and Services Offered by the National Audiovisuals Center
    Reference List of Audiovisual Materials Produced by the U.S. Government, A
    Resources in Women's Educational Equity Non-Print Media and Materials
    Selected Audiovisuals on Mental Health
    Selected Educational Media
    Selected Films: Heart Disease, Cancer, and Stroke
    Selected List: Alcohol and Drug Problems
    Source Book of Educational Materials for Radiation Therapy
    Union List of Audiovisuals in the Library Network of the Veterans Administration
    VA Film Catalog
    Video Tape Catalog Continuing Medical Education and Instruction (AHSUSA)
    Where the Drug Films Are: A Guide to Education Services and Distributors

ECOLOGY
    see ENVIRONMENTAL SCIENCES

EDUCATION
    Careers
    Special Education
    Vocational Education and Training
    see also EDUCATION, CONTINUING

    Audio-Visual Aids for High Blood Pressure Education
    Audiovisual Materials in Dental Auxiliary Education
    Cancer Film Guide
    Catalog of Audio-Visual Aids in Hypertension
    Catalog of Educational Captioned Films for the Deaf
    Catalog of the United States Coast Guard Films

EDUCATION (continued)

> Catalog of Training Films and Other Media for Special Education
> Child Abuse and Neglect Audiovisual Materials
> Criminal Justice Audiovisual Materials Directory
> Dental Training Films
> Dentistry: A Select List of U.S. Government Produced Audiovisual Materials
> Directory of Cancer Research Information Programs
> Drug Abuse Films
> Drug Abuse Prevention Films: A Multicultural Film Catalog
> Educational Media Resources in Egypt
> Energy Films Catalog
> FAA Film Catalog
> Film Archives on Child Development—The Inauguration of the Child Development Archives
> Film Catalog 1980, Pacific Region
> Film Resources on Japan
> Guide to Audio-Visual Aids for Courses in the History of Latin American Civilization in Higher Education Institutions, A
> In Focus: Alcohol and Alcoholism Media
> Indians in the United States: Select Audiovisual Records
> Library of Congress Catalogs: Audiovisual Materials
> Libros Parlantes (Talking Book Topics)
> List of Audiovisual Materials Produced by the U.S. Government for Special Education, A
> List of Audiovisual Materials Produced by the U.S. Government—Spanish Language Soundtracks, A
> Listing of Educational Materials for Use by Schools
> Medical Catalog of Selected Audiovisual Materials Produced by the U.S. Government
> Publications, Radio, Films, Slides, Fact Sheet, T.V.
> Quarterly Update: A Comprehensive Listing of New Audiovisual Materials and Services Offered by the National Audiovisual Center
> Radiological Health Training Resources Catalog
> Reference List of Audiovisual Materials Produced by the U.S. Government, A
> Selected Audiovisuals on Mental Health
> Special Education: Selected U.S. Government Audiovisuals
> Talking Book Topics
> Union List of Audiovisuals in the Library Network of the Veterans Administration
> VA Film Catalog
> Video Tape Catalog Continuing Medical Education Instruction (AHSUSA)

EDUCATION, CONTINUING
see also **EDUCATION**
RESEARCH

> Audiovisual Catalog—NIDA Resource Center
> Audiovisual Materials in Dental Auxiliary Education
> Cancer Film
> Catalog of Audio-Visual Aids in Hypertension
> Catalog of the United States Coast Guard Films
> Catalog of Training Films and Other Media for Special Education
> Child Abuse and Neglect Audiovisual Materials
> Criminal Justice Audiovisual Materials Directory

EDUCATION, CONTINUING (continued)

Dental Training Films
Directory of Cancer Research Information Resources
Drug Abuse Films
Drug Abuse Prevention Films: A Multicultural Film Catalog
Energy Films Catalog
FAA Film Catalog
Film Catalog 1980, Pacific Region
Medical Catalog of Selected Audiovisual Materials Produced by the U.S. Government
Mental Retardation Film List
NASA Film list
NIOSH—Films and Filmstrips on Occupational Safety and Health
Publications, Radio, Films, Slides, Fact Sheets, T.V.
Radiological Health Training Resources Catalog
Reference List of Audiovisual Materials Produced by the U.S. Government, A
Selected Audiovisuals on Mental Health
Union List of Audiovisuals in the Library Network of the Veterans Administration
Video Tape Catalog Continuing Medical Education and Instruction (AHSUSA)

EMBRYOLOGY

Film Guide on Reproduction and Development
Library of Congress Catalogs: Audiovisual Materials
List of Educational Aids
National Library of Medicine AVLINE Catalog
Union List of Audiovisuals in the Library Network of the Veterans Administration

EMERGENCIES

Adult Group Leader Guide for the Use with Dial A-L-C-O-H-O-L and Jackson Junior High
Army Films for Non-Profit Use
Audiovisual Aids for High Blood Pressure Education
Bimonthly List of Publications and Audiovisuals
Catalog of Films Available from Agencies: The U.S. Department of Commerce Serving the Nation
Catalog of the United States Coast Guard Films
Criminal Justice Audiovisual Materials Directory
Dental Training Films
Dentistry: A Select List of U.S. Government Produced Audiovisual Materials
Drug Abuse Prevention Films: A Multicultural Film Catalog
Federal Emergency Management Agency Motion Picture Catalog
Guide to Audiovisual Aids for Spanish-Speaking Americans
Health
In Focus: Alcohol and Alcoholism Media
Index of Army Motion Pictures for Public Non-Profit Use
Library of Congress Catalogs: Audiovisual Materials
List of Audiovisual Materials Produced by the U.S. Government in History, A
List of Audiovisual Materials Produced by the U.S. Government for Consumer Education, A
List of Audiovisual Materials Produced by the U.S. Government for Emergency Service, A

EMERGENCIES (continued)

    List of Audiovisual Materials Produced by the U.S. Government for Fire/Law Enforcement, A
    List of Audiovisual Materials Produced by the U.S. Government for Industrial Safety, A
    List of Audiovisual Materials Produced by the U.S. Government—Spanish Language Soundtracks, A
    Medical Film Catalog
    NASA Film List
    National Library of Medicine Audiovisuals Catalog
    National Library of Medicine AVLINE Catalog
    National Medical Audiovisual Center Catalog: Films for the Health Sciences
    1970 Film Reference Guide for Medicine and Allied Health Sciences
    1967 Public Health Service Film Catalog
    Publications, Radio, Films, Slides, Fact Sheets, T.V.
    Resources in Women's Educational Equity Non-Print Media and Materials
    Selected Audiovisuals on Mental Health
    Selected Educational Media
    Source Book of Educational Materials for Radiation Therapy
    Space Benefits: NASA Films and Publications Describing Benefits of Space Technology
    Training Films Mine Safety and Health Administration
    Union List of Audiovisuals in the Library Network of the Veterans Administration

ENDOCRINE SYSTEM

    List of Educational Aids
    Library of Congress Catalogs: Audiovisual Materials
    National Library of Medicine AVLINE Catalog
    Source Book of Educational Materials for Radiation Therapy

ENERGY
Conservation of Natural Resources
see also **ATOMIC ENERGY**

    Army Films for Non-Profit Use
    Bimonthly List of Publications and Audiovisuals
    Catalog of Films Available from Agencies: The U.S. Department of Commerce Serving the Nation
    Energy Efficiency Sharing: Business-to-Business Program to Facilitate Exchange of Energy Management Technology and Techniques
    Engineering: Selected U.S. Government Audiovisuals
    Energy Films Catalog
    Federal Emergency Management Agency Motion Picture Catalog
    Film Catalog
    Film Catalog 1980, Pacific Region
    Film Resources on Japan
    Forest Service Films Available on Loan to the Public for Educational Pruposes
    Library of Congress Catalogs: Audiovisual Materials
    List of Audiovisual Materials Produced by the U.S. Government for Consumer Education, A

Subject Index

ENERGY (continued)

List of Audiovisual Materials Produced by the U.S. Government for Environment and Energy Conservation, A
Medical Catalog of Selected Audiovisual Materials Produced by the U.S. Government
Medical Film Catalog
NASA Film List
Natural Resources Department Films
NIOSH—Films and Filmstrips on Occupational Safety and Health
Resource File: Practical Publications for Energy Management, The
Reference List of Audiovisual Materials Produced by the United States Government—Suppl., A
Selected Educational Media
Smithsonian Slide Series: Slides, Filmstrips. Audiocassettes. Booklets.
35 Energy Films
Union List of Audiovisuals in the Library Network of the Veterans Administration

ENGINEERING
Industry
Safety
see also OCCUPATIONAL HEALTH

Energy Films Catalog
Engineering: Selected U.S. Government Audiovisuals
Federal Emergency Management Agency Motion Picture Catalog
Films: Free from the National Bureau of Standards
Medical Catalog of Selected Audiovisual Materials Produced by the U.S. Government
NASA Film List
NIOSH—Films and Filmstrips on Occupational Safety and Health
1970 Film Reference Guide for Medicine and Allied Health Sciences
Quarterly Update: A Comprehensive Listing of New Audiovisual Materials and Services Offered by the National Audiovisual Center
Resource File: Practical Publications for Energy Management. A Reference Guide to Handbooks, Curricula, and Audiovisual Materials, The
Reference List of Audiovisual Materials Produced by the U.S. Government, A
Training Films [Mine Safety and Health Administration]

ENVIRONMENTAL HEALTH
see SAFETY
see also ENVIRONMENTAL SCIENCES

ENVIRONMENTAL SCIENCES
Bionomics
Ecology

Army Films for Non-Profit Use
Audiovisual Catalog of National Highway Traffic Safety Administration
Bimonthly List of Publications and Audiovisuals
Catalog of Films Available from Agencies: The U.S. Department of Commerce Serving the Nation
Catalog of the United States Coast Guard Films
Documentary Film Classics Produced by the U.S. Government
Educational Media Resources in Egypt

Subject Index

ENVIRONMENTAL SCIENCES (continued)

Energy Films Catalog
Engineering: Selected U.S. Government Audiovisuals
Environmental Movies and Slide Shows from EPA
Federal Emergency Management Agency Motion Picture Catalog
Film Catalog
Film Catalog 1980. Pacific Northern Region
Film Fare: A Catalog of Films and Filmstrips Produced by the U.S. Department of Housing and Urban Development
Film Resources on Japan
Films: Free from the National Bureau of Standards
Forest Service Films Available on Loan to the Public for Educational Purposes
Guide to Audio-Visual Aids for Courses in the History of Latin American Civilization in Higher Education Institutions, A
In Focus: Alcohol and Alcoholism Media
Index of Army Motion Pictures for Public Non-Profit Use
Library of Congress Catalogs: Audiovisual Materials
List of Audiovisual Materials Produced by the U.S. Government for Consumer Education, A
List of Audiovisual Materials Produced by the U.S. Government for Environment and Energy Conservation, A
List of Audiovisual Materials Produced by the U.S. Government for Industrial Safety, A
Medical Catalog of Selected Audiovisual Materials Produced by the U.S. Government
Medical Film Catalog
NASA Film List
National Library of Medicine AVLINE Catalog
Natural Resources Department Films
NIOSH—Films and Filmstrips on Occupational Safety and Health
1970 Film Reference Guide for Medicine and Allied Health Sciences
1969 Film Reference Guide for Medicine and Allied Sciences
1967 Public Health Service Film Catalog
NOAA Motion Picture Films
Recent Film Releases of the U.S. Department of Agriculture
Reference List of Audiovisual Materials Produced by the U.S. Government, A
Selected Educational Media
Resource File: Practical Publications for Energy Management. A Reference Guide to Handbooks, Curricula, and Audiovisual Materials, The
35 Energy Films
Training Films [Mine Safety and Health Administration]
Union List of Audiovisuals in the Library Network of the Veterans Administration

EPIDEMIOLOGY

Audiovisual Aids for High Blood Pressure Education
Bimonthly List of Publications and Audiovisuals
Library of Congress Catalogs: Audiovisual Materials
National Library of Medicine Audiovisuals Catalog
National Library of Medicine AVLINE Catalog
National Medical Audiovisual Center Catalog: Films for the Health Sciences
Recent Film Releases of the U.S. Department of Agriculture

EPILEPSY
see NEUROLOGY

EQUIPMENT AND SUPPLIES, MEDICAL DEVICES

Audiovisual Aids Directory of the Rehabilitation Research and Training Centers
Catalog of the FDA Publications and Audiovisual Materials for Consumers
Films: Free from the National Bureau of Standards
List of Audiovisual Materials Produced by the U.S. Government for Industrial Safety, A
Medical Cinematography
NIOSH—Films and Filmstrips on Occupational Safety and Health
Publications, Radio, Films, Slides, Fact Sheets, T.V.
Recent Film Releases of the U.S. Department of Agriculture
Training Films [Mine Safety and Health Administration]

ETHICS
see JURISPRUDENCE

ETHNIC GROUPS
see also FOREIGN LANGUAGE

Audiovisual Aids Directory of the Rehabilitation Research and Training Centers
Child Abuse and Neglect Audiovisual Materials
Film Archives on Child Development—The Inauguration of the Child Development Archives
Health: A Selected List of Books that Have Appeared in Braille Book Review, and Talking Book Topics
In Focus: Alcohol and Alcoholism Media
Selected Audiovisuals on Mental Health

EVOLUTION (Humans and Primates)
Child Development
Growth and Development
Human Development
Human Reproduction

Catalog of Family Planning Materials
Child Abuse and Neglect Audiovisual Materials
Guide to Audiovisual Aids for Spanish-Speaking Americans
Film Archives on Child Development—The Inauguration of the Child Development Archives
Film Guide on Reproduction and Development
Indians in the United States: Select Audiovisual Records
National Library of Medicine Audiovisuals Catalog
National Library of Medicine AVLINE Catalog
National Medical Audiovisual Center Catalog: Films for the Health Sciences
Smithsonian Slide Series: Slides. Filmstrips. Audiocassettes. Booklets.
Union List of Audiovisuals in the Library Network of the Veterans Administration

EXTRATERRESTRIAL ENVIRONMENT
see EXTRATERRESTRIAL ... (Miscellaneous)

Subject Index

EYE
see OPHTHALMOLOGY

FAMILY PLANNING
Birth Control
Contraceptives
Population Control

Catalog of Family Planning Materials
Catalog of Films Available from Agencies: The U.S. Department of Commerce Serving the Nation
Child Abuse and Neglect Audiovisual Materials
Film Archives on Child Development—The Inauguration of the Child Development Archives
Film Resources on Japan
Guide to Audio-Visual Aids for Courses in the History of Latin American Civilization in Higher Education Institutions, A
Guide to Audiovisual Aids for Spanish-Speaking Americans
Health
Health: A Selected List of Books that Have Appeared in Braille Book Review, and Talking Book Topics
Library of Congress Catalogs: Audiovisual Materials
List of Audiovisual Materials Produced by the U.S. Government for Social Issues, A
List of Audiovisual Materials Produced by the U.S. Government—Spanish Language Soundtracks, A
Resources in Women's Educational Equity Non-Print Media and Materials
Selected Audiovisuals on Mental Health

FATIGUE
see also PHYSICAL FITNESS
PSYCHOLOGY...
WAR
see COMBAT FATIGUE ... (Miscellaneous)

FIRST AID
see EMERGENCIES

FOOD
see also NUTRITION AND DIET

Audiovisual Guide to the Catalog of the Food and Nutrition Information and Educational Materials Center
Bimonthly List of Publications and Audiovisuals
Catalog of the FDA Publications and Audiovisual Materials for Consumers
Catalog of the United States Coast Guard Films
Documentary Film Classics Produced by the U.S. Government
Film Catalog
Film Resources on Japan
Guide to Audiovisual Aids for Spanish-Speaking Americans
Library of Congress Catalogs: Audiovisual Materials
National Library of Medicine AVLINE Catalog
Natural Resources Department Films
1970 Film Reference Guide for Medicine and Allied Health Sciences

FOOD (continued)

NOAA Motion Picture Films
Recent Film Releases of the U.S. Department of Agriculture
Union List of Audiovisuals in the Library Network of the Veterans Administration
VA Film Catalog

FOREIGN LANGUAGE
see also ETHNIC GROUPS

Audio-Visual Materials Catalog—Arthritis Information Clearinghouse
Catalog of Family Planning Materials
Catalog of the FDA Publications and Audiovisual Materials for Consumers
Child Abuse and Neglect Audiovisual Materials
Educational Media Resources in Egypt
Drug Abuse Prevention Films: A Multicultural Film Catalog
Guide to Audio-Visuals for Courses in the History of Latin American Civilization in Higher Education Institutions, A
Film Resources on Japan
Guide to Audiovisual Aids for Spanish-Speaking Americans
Health
Health: A Selected List of Books that Have Appeared in Braille Book Review, and Talking Book Topics
In Focus: Alcohol and Alcoholism Media
Libros Parlantes (Talking Book Topics)
List of Audiovisual Materials Produced by the U.S. Government for Consumer Education, A
List of Audiovisual Materials Produced by the U.S. Government for Emergency Medical Service, A
List of Audiovisual Materials Produced by the U.S. Government for Fire/Law Enforcement, A
List of Audiovisual Materials Produced by the U.S. Government for Foreign Language Instruction, A
List of Audiovisual Materials Produced by the U.S. Government for Nursing, A
List of Audiovisual Materials Produced by the U.S. Government—Spanish Language Soundtracks, A
Mental Retardation Film List
Recent Film Releases of the U.S. Department of Agriculture
Reference List of Audiovisual Materials Produced by the U.S. Government—Suppl., A
Source Book of Educational Materials for Radiation Therapy
Venereal Disease Films for the General Public

FORENSIC MEDICINE
see JURISPRUDENCE

GENETICS
Heredity

Audiovisual Aids Directory of the Rehabilitation Research and Training Centers
Catalog of Family Planning Materials
Health: A Selected List of Books that Have Appeared in Talking Book Topics and Braille Book Review

Subject Index

GENETICS (continued)

    National Library of Medicine Audiovisuals Catalog
    National Library of Medicine AVLINE Catalog
    National Medical Audiovisual Center Catalog: Films for the Health Sciences
    Source Book of Educational Materials for Radiation Therapy
    Union List of Audiovisuals in the Library Network of the Veterans Administration

GERIATRICS

    AoA Catalog of Films on Aging
    Audiovisual Aids Directory of the Rehabilitation Research and Training Centers
    Film Fare: A Catalog of Films and Filmstrips Produced by the U.S. Department of Housing and Urban Development
    Guide to Audiovisual Aids for Spanish-Speaking Americans
    Health: A Selected List of Books that Have Appeared in Braille Book Review, and Talking Book Topics
    Library of Congress Catalogs: Audiovisual Materials
    List of Audiovisual Materials Produced by the U.S. Government for Emergency Medical Service, A
    List of Audiovisual Materials Produced by the U.S. Government for Social Sciences, A
    National Library of Medicine Audiovisuals Catalog
    National Library of Medicine AVLINE Catalog
    National Medical Audiovisual Center Catalog: Films for the Health Sciences
    1970 Film Reference Guide for Medicine and Allied Health Sciences
    Radiological Health Training Resources Catalog
    Selected Audiovisuals on Mental Health
    Selected Guide to Audio-Visual Materials on Alcohol and Alcoholism, A
    Union List of Audiovisuals in the Library Network of the Veterans Administration
    VA Film Catalog

GEOLOGY
    Earth
    Moon

    Bimonthly List of Publications and Audiovisuals
    Energy Films Catalog
    Engineering: Selected U.S. Government Audiovisuals
    Environmental Movies and Slide Shows from EPA
    Film Catalog
    List of Audiovisual Materials Produced by the U.S. Government for Environment and Energy Conservation
    List of Audiovisual Materials Produced by the U.S. Government for Flight and Meteorology
    NASA Film List
    Reference List of Audiovisual Materials Produced by the U.S. Government, A
    Selected Educational Media
    Smithsonian Slide Series. Slides. Filmstrips. Audiocassettes. Booklets.
    Space Benefits: NASA Films and Publications Describing Benefits of Space and Technology
    35 Energy Films
    Viking Film Announcement

Subject Index

GOVERNMENT PROGRAMS
  see also ABUSE
        COMMUNITY HEALTH
        DRUG ABUSE
        EMERGENCIES
        PUBLIC HEALTH

    Adult Group Leader Guide for the Use with Dial A-L-C-O-H-O-L and Junior High
    AoA Catalog of Films on Aging
    Audiovisual Aids Directory of the Rehabilitation Research and Training Centers
    Audiovisual Catalog—NIDA Resource Center
    Cancer Film Guide
    Catalog of Films Available from Agencies: The U.S. Department of Commerce
        Serving the Nation
    Catalog of the FDA Publications and Audiovisual Materials for Consumers
    Catalog of the United States Coast Guard Films
    Child Abuse and Neglect Audiovisual Materials
    Dental Training Films
    Directory of Cancer Research Information Resources
    Disaster Preparedness: Publications, Films and Other Audio-Visual Materials from
        the National Weather Service
    Documentary Film Classics Produced by the United States Government
    Drug Abuse Films
    Drug Abuse Prevention Films: A Multicultural Film Catalog
    Energy Efficiency Sharing: Business-to-Business Program to Facilitate Exchange
        of Energy Management Technology and Techniques
    Energy Films Catalog
    Engineering: Selected U.S. Government Audiovisuals
    Environmental Movies and Slide Shows from EPA
    FAA Film Catalog
    Federal Emergency Management Agency Motion Picture Catalog
    Film Archives on Child Development—The Inauguration of the Child Development Archives
    Film Catalog
    Film Catalog 1980, Pacific Region
    In Focus: Alcohol and Alcoholism Media
    Index of Army Motion Pictures for Public Non-Profit Use
    List of Audiovisual Materials Produced by the U.S. Government for Business and
        Government Management, A
    List of Audiovisual Materials Produced by the U.S. Government for Consumer
        Education, A
    List of Audiovisual Materials Produced by the U.S. Government for Emergency
        Service, A
    List of Audiovisual Materials Produced by the U.S. Government for Environment
        and Energy Conservation, A
    List of Audiovisual Materials Produced by the U.S. Government for Fire/Law
        Enforcement, A
    List of Audiovisual Materials Produced by the U.S. Government for Foreign
        Language Instruction, A
    List of Audiovisual Materials Produced by the U.S. Government for Industrial
        Safety, A
    List of Audiovisual Materials Produced by the U.S. Government for Special
        Education, A

Subject Index

GOVERNMENT PROGRAMS (continued)

List of Audiovisual Materials Produced by the U.S. Government—Spanish Language Soundtracks, A
List of Audiovisual Materials Produced by the U.S. Government in History, A
Materials from the National Arts and the Handicapped Information Service: Annotated Bibliography
Medical Catalog of Selected Audiovisual Materials Produced by the U.S. Government
Media Resources Catalog
Medical Film Catalog
Motion Pictures, Films, and Audiovisual Information: Subject Bibliography
NASA Film List
NIOSH—Films and Filmstrips on Occupational Safety and Health
NOAA Motion Picture Films
Publications, Radio, Films, Slides, Fact Sheets, T.V.
Quarterly Update: A Comprehensive Listing of New Audiovisual Materials and Services Offered by the National Audiovisual Center
Radiological Health Training Resources
Recent Film Releases of the U.S. Department of Agriculture
Reference List of Audiovisual Materials Produced by the U.S. Government, A
Selected Films: Heart Disease, Cancer, and Stroke
Selected List: Alcohol and Drug Problems
Smithsonian Slide Series: Slides. Filmstrips. Audiocassettes. Booklets.
Space Benefits: NASA Films and Publications Describing Benefits of Space and Technology
Special Education: Selected U.S. Government Audiovisuals
Talking Book Topics
35 Energy Films
Where the Drug Films Are: A Guide to Evaluation Services and Distributors

HANDICAPPED
see also EDUCATION

Audiovisual Aids Directory of the Rehabilitation Research and Training Centers
Braille Book Review
Cassette Books
Catalog of Educational Captioned Films for the Deaf
Catalog of Training Films and Other Media for Special Education
Guide to Audiovisual Aids for Spanish-Speaking Americans
Health: A Selected List of Books that Have Appeared in Braille Book Review and Talking Book Topics
Library of Congress Catalogs: Audiovisual Materials
Libros Parlantes (Talking Book Topics)
List of Audiovisual Materials Produced by the U.S. Government for Business and Government Management, A
List of Audiovisual Materials Produced by the U.S. Government for Consumer Education, A
List of Audiovisual Materials Produced by the U.S. Government for Nursing, A
List of Audiovisual Materials Produced by the U.S. Government for Special Education, A
Materials from the National Arts and the Handicapped Information Service: Annotated Bibliography
Media Resources Catalog

HANDICAPPED (continued)

Neurological and Sensory Disease Film Guide
Resources in Women's Educational Equity Non-Print Media and Materials
Special Education: Selected U.S. Government Audiovisuals
Talking Book Topics
VA Film Catalog

HEALTH SERVICES
see COMMUNITY HEALTH

HEALTH RESOURCES

AoA Fact Sheet: Audiovisual Materials Sponsored by the Administration on Aging
Directory of Cancer Research Information Resources
Directory of U.S. Government Audiovisual Personnel
Where the Drug Films Are: A Guide to Evaluation Services and Distributors

HEMATOLOGY
see BLOOD

HEREDITY
see GENETICS

HISTOLOGY
see ANATOMY . . .

HISTORY OF MEDICINE

Bimonthly List of Publications and Audiovisuals
Catalog of the United States Coast Guard Films
Documentary Film Classics Produced by the U.S. Government
FAA Film Catalog
Film Archives on Child Development—The Inauguration of the Child Development Archives
Film Catalog
Health
In Focus: Alcohol and Alcoholism Media
List of Audiovisual Materials Produced by the U.S. Government in History, A
List of Educational Aids
Medical Film Catalog
NASA Film List
National Library of Medicine Audiovisuals Catalog
National Library of Medicine AVLINE Catalog
National Medical Audiovisual Center Catalog: Films for the Health Sciences
1970 Film Reference Guide for Medicine and Allied Health Sciences
NOAA Motion Picture Films
Radiological Health Resources Catalog
Reference List of Audiovisual Materials Produced by the U.S. Government, A
Selected Films: Heart Disease, Cancer, and Stroke
Smithsonian Slide Series: Slides. Filmstrips. Audiocassettes. Booklets.
Venereal Disease Films for the General Public
Viking Film Announcement

Subject Index

HOSPITALS
see HOSPITALS OVERSEAS ... (Miscellaneous)
   WAR

HYGIENE
Personal

   Army Films for Non-Profit Use
   Catalog of Educational Captioned Films for the Deaf
   Dentistry: A Select List of U.S. Government Produced Audiovisual Materials
   Guide to Audiovisual Aids for Spanish-Speaking Americans
   Health: A Selected List of Books that Have Appeared in Braille Book Review, and
      Talking Book Topics
   Index of Army Motion Pictures for Public Non-Profit Use
   NASA Film List
   VA Film Catalog

HYPERTENSION

   Audiovisual Aids for High Blood Pressure Education
   Catalog of Audio-Visual Aids in Hypertension
   Health: A Selected List of Books that Have Appeared in Talking Book Topics and
      Braille Book Review
   Guide to Audiovisual Aids for Spanish-Speaking Americans
   Library of Congress Catalogs: Audiovisual Materials
   National Library of Medicine Audiovisuals Catalog
   National Library of Medicine AVLINE Catalog
   National Medical Audiovisual Center Catalog: Films for the Health Sciences
   Quarterly Update: A Comprehensive Listing of New Audiovisual Materials and
      Services Offered by the National Audiovisual Center
   Reference List of Audiovisual Materials Produced by the U.S. Government, A
   Selected Films: Heart Disease, Cancer, and Stroke
   Union List of Audiovisuals in the Library Network of the Veterans Administration

INDIANS
see MINORITY GROUPS

   Indians in the United States: Select Audiovisual Records

INDUSTRIAL HYGIENE
see OCCUPATIONAL HEALTH

INFECTIOUS DISEASES
see COMMUNICABLE DISEASES

JURISPRUDENCE
Criminal Law
Ethics
Forensic Medicine

   Adult Group Leader Guide for the Use with Dial A-L-C-O-H-O-L and Jackson
      Junior High
   Audiovisual Materials in Dental Auxiliary Education

JURISPRUDENCE (continued)

    Audiovisual Catalog of the National Highway Traffic Safety Administration
    Audiovisual Catalog—NIDA Resource Center
    Audio Visual Materials Catalog—Arthritis Information Clearinghouse
    Catalog of Films Available from Agencies: The U.S. Department of Commerce Serving the Nation
    Child Abuse and Neglect Audiovisual Materials
    Criminal Justice Audiovisual Materials Directory
    Documentary Film Classics Produced by the U.S. Government
    Drug Abuse Films
    Drug Abuse Prevention Films: A Multicultural Film Catalog
    Environmental Movies and Slide Shows from EPA
    Films: Free from the National Bureau of Standards
    In Focus: Alcohol and Alcoholism Media
    Library of Congress Catalogs: Audiovisual Materials
    List of Audiovisual Materials Produced by the U.S. Government for Consumer Education, A
    List of Audiovisual Materials Produced by the U.S. Government for Fire/Law Enforcement, A
    List of Educational Aids
    Reference List of Audiovisual Materials Produced by the United States Government—Suppl., A
    Media Resources Catalog
    1970 Film Reference Guide for Medicine and Allied Health Sciences
    Publications, Radio, Films, Slides, Fact Sheets, T.V.
    Quarterly Update: A Comprehensive Listing of New Audiovisual Materials and Services Offered by the National Audiovisual Center
    Selected Audiovisuals on Mental Health
    Selected Guide to Audio-Visual Materials on Alcohol and Alcoholism, A
    Source Book of Educational Materials for Radiation Therapy
    Training Films [Mine Safety and Health Administration]
    Union List of Audiovisuals in the Library Network of the Veterans Administration

LABORATORIES

    Energy Films Catalog
    Film Catalog 1980, Pacific Region
    Index to Army Motion Pictures for Public Non-Profit Use
    List of Educational Aids
    List of Audiovisual Materials Produced by the U.S. Government for Industrial Safety, A
    Medical Film Catalog
    National Library of Medicine AVLINE Catalog
    NIOSH—Films and Filmstrips on Occupational Safety and Health Filmstrips
    NOAA Motion Picture Films
    Source Book of Educational Materials for Radiation Therapy
    Space Benefits: NASA Films and Publications Describing Benefits of Space and Technology
    Training Films [Mine Safety and Health Administration]

Subject Index

LANGUAGE
see **FOREIGN LANGUAGE**

LASERS
see also **RADIOLOGY**
TECHNOLOGY

 List of Educational Aids

LIBRARY SCIENCES
see also **TECHNOLOGY**

 Medical Catalog of Selected Audiovisual Materials Produced by the U.S. Government
 Problems in Bibliographic Access to Non-Print Materials, Project Media Base: Final Report

MANAGEMENT
see **ORGANIZATION AND ADMINISTRATION**

MARINE BIOLOGY
see **MARINE SCIENCES**

MARINE SCIENCES
Marine Biology
Oceanography
Submarine Medicine

 Bimonthly List of Publications and Audiovisuals
 Career Education: Selected U.S. Government Audiovisuals
 Catalog of Films Available from Agencies: The U.S. Department of Commerce Serving the Nation
 Catalog of the United States Coast Guard
 Disaster Preparedness: Publications, Films and Other Audio-Visual Materials from the National Weather Service
 Engineering: Selected U.S. Government Audiovisuals
 Film Catalog
 Library of Congress Catalogs: Audiovisual Materials
 Medical Film Catalog
 NOAA Motion Picture Films
 Reference List of Audiovisual Materials Produced by the United States Government—Suppl., A
 Space Benefits: NASA Films and Publications Describing Benefits of Space Technology

MATHEMATICS

 Catalog of Educational Captioned Films for the Deaf

MEN AND WOMEN

 Indians in the United States: Select Audiovisual Records
 List of Educational Aids
 Resources in Women's Educational Equity Non-Print Media and Materials

Subject Index

MENTAL HEALTH
Behavior Modification

Adult Group Leader for the Use with Dial A-L-C-O-H-O-L and Jackson Junior High
Audiovisual Aids Directory of the Rehabilitation Research and Training Centers
Audiovisual Catalog—NIDA Resource Center
Child Abuse and Neglect Audiovisual Materials
Criminal Justice Audiovisual Materials Directory
Guide to Audiovisual Aids for Spanish-Speaking Americans
Library of Congress Catalogs: Audiovisual Materials
List of Audiovisual Materials Produced by the U.S. Government for Nursing, A
List of Audiovisual Materials Produced by the U.S. Government for Social Sciences, A
Media Resources Catalog
Mental Retardation Film List
National Library of Medicine Audiovisuals Catalog
National Medical Audiovisual Center Catalog: Films for the Health Sciences
Reference List of Audiovisual Materials Produced by the U.S. Government, A
Resources in Women's Educational Equity Non-Print Media and Materials
Selected Audiovisuals on Mental Health
Selected Guide to Audio Visual Materials on Alcohol and Alcoholism, A
Selected List: Alcohol and Drug Problems
Video Tape Catalog Continuing Medical Education and Instruction (AHSUSA)

MENTAL RETARDATION
see also MENTAL HEALTH

Audiovisual Aids Directory of the Rehabilitation Research and Training Centers
Child Abuse and Neglect Audiovisual Materials
Guide to Audiovisual Aids for Spanish-Speaking Americans, A
List of Audiovisual Materials Produced by the U.S. Government for Special Education, A
List of Audiovisual Materials Produced by the U.S. Government for Nursing, A
Mental Retardation Film List
National Library of Medicine Audiovisuals Catalog
Neurological and Sensory Disease Film Guide
Selected Audiovisuals on Mental Health
Special Education: Selected U.S. Government Audiovisuals

METEOROLOGY
see CLIMATE . . .

METRIC SYSTEM

Audiovisual Guide to the Catalog of the Food and Nutrition Information and Educational Materials Center
Catalog of Films Available from Agencies: The United States Department of Commerce Serving the Nation
Source Book of Educational Materials for Radiation Therapy

Subject Index

MICROBIOLOGY

    National Library of Medicine Audiovisuals Catalog
    National Library of Medicine AVLINE Catalog
    National Medical Audiovisual Center Catalog: Films for the Health Sciences

MILITARY MEDICINE

    Documentary Film Classics Produced by the U.S. Government
    Index of Army Motion Pictures for Public Non-Profit Use
    List of Audiovisual Materials Produced by the U.S. Government for Emergency Medical Service, A
    List of Educational Aids
    Medical Catalog of Selected Audiovisual Materials Produced by the U.S. Government
    Medical Film Catalog
    National Library of Medicine Audiovisuals Catalog
    Nationsl Library of Medicine AVLINE Catalog
    National Medical Audiovisual Center Catalog: Films for the Health Sciences
    Selected Educational Media
    Union List of Audiovisuals in the Library Network of the Veterans Administration
    VA Film Catalog
    Video Tape Catalog Continuing Medical Education and Instruction (AHSUSA)

MINING

    List of Audiovisual Materials Produced by the U.S. Government for Industrial Safety, A
    NIOSH—Films and Filmstrips on Occupational Safety and Health
    Training Films [Mine Safety and Health Administration]

MINORITY GROUPS (including American Indians)
  Culture
  see also **FOREIGN LANGUAGE**

    Child Abuse and Neglect Audiovisual Materials
    Drug Abuse Prevention Films: A Multicultural Film Catalog
    In Focus: Alcohol and Alcoholism Media
    List of Audiovisual Materials Produced by the U.S. Government for Social Sciences, A
    List of Audiovisual Materials Produced by the U.S. Government—Spanish Language Soundtracks, A
    Libros Parlantes (Talking Book Topics)
    Selected Audiovisuals on Mental Health
    Selected Guide to Audio-Visual Materials on Alcohol and Alcoholism, A
    Union List of Audiovisuals in the Library Network of the Veterans Administration

MISCELLANEOUS

  Abstracts
    Directory of Cancer Research Information Resources

  AMA Studies on Accidents and their Causes
    Audiovisual Catalog of National Highway Traffic and Safety Administration

MISCELLANEOUS (continued)

AMVER (Automated Mutual-Assistance Vessel Rescue System)
Catalog of the United States Coast Guard Films

Arts
Reference List of Audiovisual Materials Produced by the U.S. Government, A

Baby Sitters
Listing of Educational Materials for Use by Schools

Bionomics
Film Catalog
Guide to Audio-Visual Aids for Courses in the History of Latin American Civilization in Higher Education, A

Cartier-Bresson, Henri
Documentary Film Classics

Chemical, Biological, and Radiological Warfare
Army Films for Non-Profit Use
Index of Army Motion Pictures for Public Non Profit Use
Reference List of Audiovisual Materials Produced by the United States Government—Suppl., A

Cinematography
Medical Cinematography

Combat Fatigue—Traumatic Neurosis
Army Films for Non-Profit Use
Index to Army Motion Pictures for Public Non-Profit Use
Union List of Audiovisual Materials in the Library Network of the Veterans Administration
VA Film Catalog

Capra, Frank
Documentary Film Classics

CPR (Cardiopulmonary Resuscitation)
List of Audiovisual Materials Produced by the U.S. Government for Emergency Medical Service, A
List of Audiovisual Materials Produced by the U.S. Government—Spanish Language Soundtracks, A
Source Book of Educational Materials for Radiation Therapy

Creativity
Catalog of Training Films and Other Media for Special Education

Crimes Against Humanity
List of Audiovisual Materials Produced by the U.S. Government in History, A

Subject Index

MISCELLANEOUS (continued)

DIAL A-L-C-O-H-O-L Series
    Adult Group Leader Guide for the Use with DIAL A-L-C-O-H-O-L and Junior High
    Audiovisual Catalog—NIDA Resource Center

Disorientation
    List of Audiovisual Materials Produced by the U.S. Government for Flight and Meteorology

Documents
    Directory of Cancer Research Information Resources

Einstein's Theory
    Smithsonian Slide Series: Slides. Filmstrips. Audiocassettes. Booklets.

Extraterrestrial Life
    Viking Film Announcement

Fermi Laboratory—Discovery of Plutonium
    List of Audiovisual Materials Produced by the U.S. Government in History, A

Firearms
    Natural Resources Department Films

Flaherty, J. Robert
    Documentary Film Classics

Ford, John
    Documentary Film Classics

Gesell, Arnold
    Film Archives for Child Development—The Inauguration of the Child Development Archives

Grayson, Helen
    Documentary Film Classics

Hammid, Alexander
    Documentary Film Classics

Heat Stroke
    Index to Army Motion Pictures for Public Non-Profit Use

Herpetology
    Bimonthly List of Publications and Audiovisuals

Hiroshima/Nagasaki
    List of Audiovisual Materials Produced by the U.S. Government in History, A
    Film Resources of Japan

MISCELLANEOUS (continued)

Horticultural Society
    Natural Resources Department Films

Hospitals Overseas During Wars—WWI, II, Viet Nam
    Army Films for Non-Profit Use
    Documentary Film Classics Produced by the U.S. Government
    Index of Army Motion Pictures for Non-Profit Use
    List of Audiovisual Materials Produced by the U.S. Government in History, A

Huston, John
    Documentary Film Classics

Hyperactivity
    Audiovisual Aids Directory of the Rehabilitation Research and Training Centers

Hypnosis
    Union List of Audiovisual Materials in the Library Network of the Veterans Administration

Hypoxia
    Audiovisual Aids Directory of the Rehabilitation Research and Training Centers
    List of Audiovisual Materials Produced by the U.S. Government for Flight and Meteorology, A

Imprisonment
    Criminal Justice Audiovisual Materials Directory
    Documentary Film Classics Produced by the U.S. Government
    Drug Abuse Films
    Media Resources Catalog

Ivens, Joris
    Documentary Film Classics

Kanin, Garson
    Documentary Film Classics

Lerner, Irving
    Documentary Film Classics

Life—Hypothetical Conclusions of Type of Possible Life Forms
    Viking Film Announcement

Livingston, Dr.—Life and Work of Dr. David Livingston
    Educational Media Resources on Egypt

Lorentz, Pare
    Documentary Film Classics

Mahler, Margaret
    Film Archives for Child Development—The Inauguration of the Child Development Archives

Subject Index

MISCELLANEOUS (continued)

McMechen, Jervis B.
Documentary Film Classics

Medical Teamwork of the U.S. Army Environmental Hygiene Agency
Index to Army Motion Pictures for Public Non-Profit Use

Medical Terminology
Source Book of Educational Materials for Radiation Therapy

Medicine for the Laymen
Health

Montessori
Catalog of Training Films and Other Media for Special Education

Mutual of Omaha—"Wild Kingdom" Series
Film Catalog

NASTRAN (Solving Structural Engineering Design Problems in Industry)
NASA Film List
Space Benefits: NASA Films and Publications Describing Benefits of Space and Technology

Nevada Test Site
35 Energy Films

Personnel—Audiovisual
Directory of U.S. Audiovisual Personnel

Piaget
Catalog of Training Films and Other Media for Special Education

Pictorial Atlas to Tumor Pathology
List of Educational Aids

Polar Medicine
Media Resources Catalog

Prescription Writing
Audiovisual Materials in Dental Auxiliary Education

Reed, Carol
Documentary Film Classics

Sailing—Safety
Natural Resources Department of Films

Sierra Club, The
Environmental Movies and Slide Shows from EPA

MISCELLANEOUS (continued)

Sleeping Sickness
Bimonthly List of Publications and Audiovisuals

Spewack, Samuel
Documentary Film Classics

Sponge Industry, The
Catalog of Films Available from Agencies: The United States Department of Commerce Serving the Nation

Stone, L. Joseph
Film Archives for Child Development—The Inauguration of the Child Development Archives

Submarine—Ocean Instrumentation
Engineering: Selected U.S. Government Audiovisuals

Surgical Removal of Scars on Prisoners
Criminal Justice Audiovisual Materials Directory

Technology (Special)—GARP (Global Atlantic Research Programs)—GATE (Atlantic Tropical Experiment), NISS (National Injury Surveillance System)
NOAA Motion Picture Films
Publications, Radio, Films, Slides, Fact Sheets, T.V.

Terradynamics
Engineering: Selected U.S. Government Audiovisuals

Three Mile Island
Radiological Health Training Resources Catalog

U.S. Counsel for the Prosecution of Axis Criminality
Documentary Film Classics

Van Dyke, Willard
Documentary Film Classics

Venipuncture
Audiovisual Materials in Dental Auxiliary Education

Violence (Body)
Criminal Justice Audiovisual Materials Directory

von Sternberg, Joseph
Documentary Film Classics

Waggner, George
Documentary Film Classics

Subject Index

MISCELLANEOUS (continued)

Walt Disney—Classic Health Series
Guide to Audiovisual Aids for Spanish-Speaking Americans, A
Health: Selected List of Books that Have Appeared in Talking Book Topics and Braille Book Review
Health

"War of the Worlds," The—Orson Welles' 1938 Radio Broadcast
Viking Film Announcement

Welles, Orson, "The War of the Worlds," 1938 Radio Broadcast
Viking Film Announcement

WHO (Work of Pan American Health Organization)
Library of Congress Catalogs

Wright Brothers, The
FAA Film Catalog

Wyler, William
Documentary Film Classics

MUSCULOSKELETAL SYSTEM

Library of Congress Catalogs: Audiovisual Materials
National Library of Medicine Audiovisuals Catalog
National Library of Medicine AVLINE Catalog
National Medical Audiovisual Center Catalog: Films for the Health Sciences
Union List of Audiovisuals in the Library Network of the Veterans Administration
VA Film Catalog

NAVAL MEDICINE
see MARINE SCIENCES

NEOPLASMS

Audiovisual Aids Directory of the Rehabilitation Research and Training Centers
Audiovisual Materials in Dental Auxiliary Education
Cancer Film Guide
Catalog of Family Planning Materials
Dentistry: A Select List of U.S. Government Produced Audiovisual Materials
Directory of Cancer Research Information Resources
Guide to Audiovisual Aids for Spanish-Speaking Americans
Library of Congress Catalogs: Audiovisual Materials
National Library of Medicine Audiovisuals Catalog
National Library of Medicine AVLINE Catalog
National Medical Audiovisual Center Catalog: Films for the Health Sciences
1970 Film Reference Guide for Medicine and Allied Health Sciences
1969 Film Reference Guide for Medicine and Allied Sciences
1967 Public Health Service Film Catalog
Reference List of Audiovisual Materials Produced by the U.S. Government, A
Selected Films: Heart Disease, Cancer, and Stroke

NEOPLASMS (continued)

Source Book of Educational Materials for Radiation Therapy
Union List of Audiovisuals in the Library Network of the Veterans Administation
VA Film Catalog
Video Tape Catalog Continuing Education and Instruction (AHSUSA)

NEUROLOGY

Audiovisual Aids Directory of the Rehabilitation Research and Training Centers
Guide to Audiovisual Aids for Spanish-Speaking Americans
List of Educational Aids
Medical Film Catalog
National Library of Medicine Audiovisuals Catalog
National Medical Audiovisual Center Catalog: Films for the Health Sciences
Neurological and Sensory Disease Film Guide
Selected Audiovisuals on Mental Health
Source Book of Educational Materials for Radiation Therapy
Union List of Audiovisuals in the Library Network of the Veterans Administration
VA Film Catalog

NUCLEAR MEDICINE
see **NUCLEAR SCIENCES**

NUCLEAR SCIENCES
Nuclear Medicine

Army Films for Non-Profit Use
Energy Films Catalog
Engineering: Selected U.S. Government Audiovisuals
Index of Army Motion Pictures for Public Non-Profit Use
Medical Film Catalog
Smithsonian Slide Series: Slides. Filmstrips. Audiocassettes. Booklets.
List of Audiovisual Materials Produced by the U.S. Government in History, A
List of Audiovisual Materials Produced by the U.S. Government for Emergency Medical Service, A
Radiological Health Training Resources Catalog
Source Book of Educational Materials for Radiation Therapy
35 Energy Films

NURSING

Army Films for Non-Profit Use
Audiovisual Aids Directory of the Rehabilitation Research and Training Centers
Audiovisual Aids for High Blood Pressure
Child Abuse and Neglect Audiovisual Materials
Dentistry: A Select List of U.S. Government Produced Audiovisual Materials
Directory of Cancer Research Information Programs
Film Fare: A Catalog of Films and Filmstrips Produced by the U.S. Department of Housing and Urban Development
Index of Army Motion Pictures for Public Non-Profit Use
List of Audiovisual Materials Produced by the U.S. Government in History, A
List of Audiovisual Materials Produced by the U.S. Government for Nursing, A

Subject Index

NURSING (continued)

List of Educational Aids
Library of Congress Catalogs: Audiovisual Materials
Medical Catalog of Selected Audiovisual Materials Produced by the U.S. Government
National Library of Medicine Audiovisuals Catalog
National Library of Medicine AVLINE Catalog
National Medical Audiovisual Center Catalog: Films for the Health Sciences
NIOSH—Films and Filmstrips on Occupational Safety and Health
1970 Film Reference Guide for Medicine and Allied Health Sciences
1969 Film Reference Guide for Medicine and Allied Sciences
1967 Public Health Service Film Catalog
Reference List of Audiovisual Materials Produced by the U.S. Government, A
Resources in Women's Educational Equity Non-Print Media and Materials
Source Book of Educational Materials for Radiation Therapy
Union List of Audiovisuals in the Library Network of the Veterans Administration
VA Film Catalog
Video Tape Catalog Continuing Medical Education and Instruction (AHSUSA)

NUTRITION AND DIET
see also FOOD

AoA Catalog of Films on Aging
Audiovisual Aids for High Blood Pressure Education
Audiovisual Guide to the Catalog of the Food and Nutrition Information and Educational Materials Center
Audio Visual Materials Catalog—Arthritis Information Clearinghouse
Audiovisual Materials in Dental Auxiliary Education
Bimonthly List of Publications and Audiovisuals
Child Abuse and Neglect Audiovisual Materials
Film Resources on Japan
Guide to Audiovisual Aids for Spanish-Speaking Americans
Health: A Selected List of Books that Have Appeared in Braille Book Review, and Talking Book Topics
In Focus: Alcohol and Alcoholism Media
List of Audiovisual Materials Produced by the U.S. Government—Spanish Language Soundtracks, A
List of Educational Aids
Medical Catalog of Selected Audiovisual Materials Produced by the U.S. Government
1970 Film Reference Guide for Medicine and Allied Health Sciences
1967 Public Health Services Film Catalog
NOAA Motion Picture Films
VA Film Catalog

OBSTETRICS/GYNECOLOGY

Army Films for Non-Profit Use
Audiovisual Aids for High Blood Pressure Education
Audiovisual Guide to the Catalog of the Food and Nutrition Information and Educational Materials Center
Educational Media Resources on Egypt
Film Guide on Reproduction and Development
Guide to Audiovisual Aids for Spanish-Speaking Americans

Subject Index

OBSTETRICS/GYNECOLOGY (continued)

    Health: A Selected List of Books that Have Appeared in Braille Book Review, and Talking Book Topics
    List of Audiovisual Materials Produced by the U.S. Government for Emergency Medical Services, A
    Medical Film Catalog
    National Library of Medicine Audiovisuals Catalog
    National Medical Audiovisual Center Catalog: Films for the Health Sciences
    1970 Film Reference Guide for Medicine and Allied Health Sciences
    1969 Film Reference Guide for Medicine and Allied Sciences
    1967 Public Health Service Film Catalog
    Resources in Women's Educational Equity Non-Print Media and Materials
    Video Tape Catalog Continuing Medical Education and Instruction (AHSUSA)

OCCUPATIONAL HEALTH
  Occupational Medicine
  Preventive Medicine

    AoA Catalog of Films on Aging
    Army Films for Non-Profit Use
    Audio Visual Materials Catalog—Arthritis Information Clearinghouse
    Audiovisual Guide to the Catalog of Food and Nutrition Information and Educational Materials Guide
    Audiovisual Materials in Dental Auxiliary Education
    Dental Training Films
    Dentistry: A Select List of U.S. Government Produced Audiovisual Materials
    Directory of Cancer Research Information Resources
    Documentary Film Classics Produced by the U.S. Government
    Drug Abuse Prevention Films: A Multicultural Film Catalog
    Engineering: Selected U.S. Government Audiovisuals
    Films: Free from the National Bureau of Standards
    Health
    Guide to Audiovisual Aids for Spanish-Speaking Americans
    In Focus: Alcohol and Alcoholism Media
    Index of Army Motion Pictures for Public Non-Profit Use
    Library of Congress Catalogs: Audiovisual Materials
    List of Audiovisual Materials Produced by the U.S. Government for Business and Government Personnel, A
    List of Audiovisual Materials Produced by the U.S. Government for Industrial Safety, A
    Medical Catalog of Selected Audiovisual Materials Produced by the U.S. Government
    Medical Film Catalog
    National Library of Medicine Audiovisuals Catalog
    National Library of Medicine AVLINE Catalog
    National Medical Audiovisual Center Catalog: Films for the Health Sciences
    1969 Film Reference Guide for Medicine and Allied Sciences
    1967 Public Health Service Film Catalog
    NIOSH—Films and Filmstrips on Occupational Safety and Health
    Reference List of Audiovisual Materials Produced by the United States Government—Suppl., A
    Resources in Women's Educational Equity Non-Print Media and Materials
    Selected Films: Heart Disease, Cancer, and Stroke

OCCUPATIONAL HEALTH (continued)

 Space Benefits: NASA Films and Publications Describing Benefits of Space Technology
 Training Films [Mine Safety and Health Administration]
 Union List of Audiovisuals in the Library Network of the Veterans Administration
 VA Film Catalog

OCCUPATIONAL MEDICINE
 see OCCUPATIONAL HEALTH

OCCUPATIONAL THERAPY
 see PHYSICAL THERAPY

OCEANOGRAPHY
 see MARINE SCIENCES

OPHTHALMOLOGY

 Health: A Selected List of Books that Have Appeared in Braille, and Talking Book Topics
 Catalog of Training Films and Other Media for Special Education
 List of Audiovisual Materials Produced by the U.S. Government for Flight and Meteorology
 Medical Cinematography
 Medical Film Catalog
 National Library of Medicine Audiovisuals Catalog
 National Library of Medicine AVLINE Catalog
 National Medical Audiovisual Center Catalog: Films for the Health Sciences
 Neurological and Sensory Disease Film Guide
 NIOSH—Films and Filmstrips on Occupational Safety and Health
 Reference List of Audiovisual Materials Produced by the U.S. Government, A
 Union List of Audiovisuals in the Library Network of the Veterans Administration

ORGANIZATION AND ADMINISTRATION
Business and Economics
Management

 Audiovisual Materials in Dental Auxiliary Education
 Child Abuse and Neglect Audiovisual Materials
 FAA Film Catalog
 Medical Film Catalog
 National Library of Medicine AVLINE Catalog
 Quarterly Update: A Comprehensive Listing of New Audiovisual Materials and Services Offered by the National Audiovisual Center
 Reference List of Audiovisual Materials Produced by the U.S. Government, A
 Union List of Audiovisuals in the Library Network of the Veterans Administration
 VA Film Catalog

ORTHOPEDICS

 List of Educational Aids
 Medical Film Catalog

ORTHOPEDICS (continued)

1969 Film Reference Guide for Medicine and Allied Sciences
Union List of Audiovisuals in the Library Network of the Veterans Administration
VA Film Catalog

OTORHINOLARYNGOLOGY

Army Films for Non-Profit Use
Catalog of Training Films and Other Media for Special Education
Library of Congress Catalogs: Audiovisual Materials
List of Educational Aids
Medical Cinematography
Medical Film Catalog
National Library of Medicine Audiovisuals Catalog
National Library of Medicine AVLINE Catalog
National Medical Audiovisual Center Catalog: Films for the Health Sciences
Neurological and Sensory Disease Film Guide
1969 Film Reference Guide for Medicine and Allied Sciences
Union List of Audiovisuals in the Library Network of the Veterans Administration
Video Tape Catalog Continuing Medical Education and Instruction (AHSUSA)

PATHOLOGY

Audiovisual Materials in Dental Auxiliary Education
Dental Training Films
Film Archives on Child Development—The Inauguration of the Child Development Archives
List of Educational Aids
Medical Film Catalog
Selected Films: Heart Disease, Cancer, and Stroke

PATIENT EDUCATION

Audiovisual Materials in Dental Auxiliary Education
Catalog of Audio-Visual Aids in Hypertension
Catalog of Training Films and Other Media for Special Education
Dental Training Films
Dentistry: A Select List of U.S. Government Produced Audiovisual Materials
Drug Abuse Films
Health
In Focus: Alcohol and Alcoholism Media
Medical Film Catalog
Radiological Health Training Resources Catalog
Selected Films: Heart Disease, Cancer, and Stroke
Selected List: Alcohol and Drug Problems
Source Book of Educational Materials for Radiation Therapy
Talking Book Topics
Venereal Disease Films for the General Public
VA Film Catalog

Subject Index

PEDIATRICS

    Audiovisual Guide to the Catalog of the Food and Nutrition Information and Educational Materials Center
    Child Abuse and Neglect Audiovisual Materials
    Library of Congress Catalogs: Audiovisuals Materials
    List of Educational Aids
    Medical Film Catalog
    National Library of Medicine Audiovisuals Catalog
    National Library of Medicine AVLINE Catalog
    National Medical Audiovisual Center Catalog: Films for the Health Sciences
    Union List of Audiovisuals in the Library Network of the Veterans Administration

PERSONNEL
    see PERSONNEL . . . (Miscellaneous)

PESTICIDES
  see also CHEMISTRY . . .
      ENVIRONMENTAL SCIENCES
      POISONING
      TOXICOLOGY

    Audiovisual Guide to the Catalog of the Food and Nutrition Information and Educational Materials Center
    Bimonthly List of Publications and Audiovisuals
    Film Catalog
    Index of Army Motion Pictures for Public Non-Profit Use
    List of Audiovisual Materials Produced by the U.S. Government for Environment and Energy Conservation, A
    List of Audiovisual Materials Produced by the U.S. Government—Spanish Language Soundtracks, A
    NIOSH—Films and Filmstrips on Occupational Safety and Health
    Recent Film Releases of the U.S. Department of Agriculture

PHYSIOLOGY
    see ANATOMY

PHYSICAL FITNESS, RECREATION, SPORTS

    Audiovisual Aids Directory of the Rehabilitation Research and Training Centers
    Bimonthly List of Publications and Audiovisuals
    Catalog of Films Available from Agencies: The U.S. Department of Commerce Serving the Nation
    Catalog of the United States Coast Guard Films
    Catalog of Training Films and Other Media for Special Education
    Film Fare: A Catalog of Films and Filmstrips Produced by the U.S. Department of Housing and Urban Development
    Film Resources on Japan
    Forest Service Films Available on Loan to the Public for Educational Purposes
    Guide to Audiovisual Aids for Spanish-Speaking Americans
    Health
    Health: A Selected List of Books that Have Appeared in Talking Book Topics, and Braille Book Review

PHYSICAL FITNESS, RECREATION, SPORTS (continued)

Library of Congress Catalogs: Audiovisual Materials
List of Audiovisual Materials Produced by the U.S. Government for Business and Government Personnel, A
List of Audiovisual Materials Produced by the U.S. Government for Consumer Education, A
List of Audiovisual Materials Produced by the U.S. Government for Emergency Service, A
Medical Catalog of Selected Audiovisual Materials Produced by the U.S. Government
National Library of Medicine Audiovisuals Catalog
National Library of Medicine AVLINE Catalog
National Medical Audiovisual Center Catalog: Films for the Health Sciences
Recent Film Releases of the U.S. Department of Agriculture
Reference List of Audiovisual Materials Produced by the U.S. Government, A
Resources in Women's Educational Equity Non-Print Media and Materials
Union List of Audiovisuals in the Library Network of the Veterans Administration
VA Film Catalog

PHYSICAL MEDICINE

Audiovisual Aids Directory of the Rehabilitation Research and Training Centers
Medical Film Catalog
National Library of Medicine Audiovisuals Catalog
National Medical Audiovisual Center Catalog: Films for the Health Sciences
Smithsonian Slide Series: Slides. Filmstrips. Audiocassettes. Booklets.

PHYSICAL THERAPY, OCCUPATIONAL THERAPY

Army Films for Non-Profit Use
Index of Army Films for Non-Profit Use
Library of Congress Catalogs: Audiovisual Materials
List of Audiovisual Materials Produced by the U.S. Government for Business and Government Management, A
List of Educational Aids
Medical Film Catalog
National Library of Medicine Audiovisuals Catalog
National Library of Medicine AVLINE Catalog
National Medical Audiovisual Center Catalog: Films for the Health Sciences
1969 Film Reference Guide for Medicine and Allied Sciences
Union List of Audiovisuals in the Library Network of the Veterans Administration
VA Film Catalog

PHYSICS

Energy Films Catalog
Engineering: Selected U.S. Government Audiovisuals
Reference List of Audiovisual Materials Produced by the United States Government, A
Smithsonian Slide Series: Slides. Filmstrips. Audiocassettes. Booklets.
Source Book of Educational Materials for Radiation Therapy

Subject Index

PLANTS
see AGRICULTURE

POISONING
see also TOXICOLOGY

    Audiovisuals Guide to the Catalog of the Food and Nutrition Information and Educational Materials Center
Catalog of Films Available from Agencies: The U.S. Department of Commerce Serving the Nation
Engineering: Selected Government Audiovisuals
Film Catalog
Films: Free from the National Bureau of Standards
List of Audiovisual Materials Produced by the U.S. Government for Industrial Safety, A
Listing of Educational Materials for Use by Schools
National Library of Medicine Audiovisuals Catalog
National Library of Medicine AVLINE Catalog
National Medical Audiovisual Center Catalog: Films for the Health Sciences
NIOSH—Films and Filmstrips on Occupational Safety and Health
Publications, Radio, Films, Slides, Fact Sheets, T.V.
Recent Film Releases of the U.S. Department of Agriculture
Reference List of Audiovisual Materials Produced by the U.S. Government, A

POPULATION CONTROL
see FAMILY PLANNING

PREVENTIVE MEDICINE
see OCCUPATIONAL HEALTH

PRISONS
Concentration Camps
Prison Hospitals
see also IMPRISONMENT . . . (Miscellaneous)

    Criminal Justice Audiovisual Materials Directory
Documentary Film Classics Produced by the U.S. Government
List of Audiovisual Materials Produced by the U.S. Government in History, A
Media Resource Catalog
Medical Film Catalog

PUBLIC HEALTH
see also COMMUNITY HEALTH

    Audiovisual Aids Directory of the Rehabilitation Research and Training Centers
Cancer Film Guide
Child Abuse and Neglect Audiovisual Materials
Criminal Justice Audiovisual Materials Directory
Directory of Cancer Research Information Resources
Drug Abuse Films
Drug Abuse Prevention Films: A Multicultural Film Catalog
Energy Films Catalog
Environmental Movies and Slide Shows from EPA

PUBLIC HEALTH (continued)

    Film Fare: A Catalog of Films and Filmstrips Produced by the U.S. Department of Housing and Urban Development
    In Focus: Alcohol and Alcoholism Media
    List of Audiovisual Materials Produced by the U.S. Government for Business and Government Personnel, A
    Media Resources Catalog
    Mental Retardation Film List
    National Library of Medicine Audiovisuals Catalog
    National Library of Medicine AVLINE Catalog
    National Medical Audiovisual Cneter Catalog: Films for the Health Sciences
    NIOSH—Films and Filmstrips on Occupational Safety and Health
    Publications, Radio, Films, Slides, Fact Sheets, T.V.
    Selected Films: Heart Disease, Cancer, and Stroke
    Selected List: Alcohol and Drug Problems
    Space Benefits: NASA Films and Publications Describing Benefits of Space and Technology
    Talking Book Topics
    Training Films [Mine Safety and Health Administration]
    Union List of Audiovisuals in the Library Network of the Veterans Administration
    VA Film Catalog

PULMONARY

    Audiovisual Aids Directory of the Rehabilitation Research and Training Centers
    National Library of Medicine Audiovisuals Catalog
    National Library of Medicine AVLINE Catalog
    National Medical Audiovisual Center Catalog: Films for the Health Sciences
    Selected Films: Heart Disease, Cancer, and Stroke
    Training Films [Mine Safety and Health Administration]

PSYCHIATRY and PSYCHOLOGY

    Adult Group Leader Guide for the Use with Dial A-L-C-O-H-O-L and Jackson Junior High
    Audiovisual Aids Directory of the Rehabilitation Research and Training Centers
    Catalog of Training Films and Other Media for Special Education
    Child Abuse and Neglect Audiovisual Materials
    Criminal Justice Audiovisual Materials Directory
    Documentary Film Classics Produced by the U.S. Government
    Drug Abuse Films
    Drug Abuse Prevention Films: A Multicultural Film Catalog
    Film Archives on Child Development—The Inauguration of the Child Development Archives
    In Focus: Alcohol and Alcoholism Media
    Index of Army Motion Pictures for Public Non-Profit Use
    List of Audiovisual Materials Produced by the U.S. Government for Flight and Meteorology, A
    List of Audiovisual Materials Produced by the U.S. Government for Social Sciences, A
    List of Audiovisual Materials Produced by the U.S. Government—Spanish Language Soundtracks, A

Subject Index

PSYCHIATRY and PSYCHOLOGY (continued)

    Media Resources Catalog
    Medical Film Catalog
    Mental Retardation Film List
    Library of Congress Catalogs: Audiovisual Materials
    National Library of Medicine Audiovisuals Catalog
    National Library of Medicine AVLINE Catalog
    National Medical Audiovisual Center Catalog: Films for the Health Sciences
    1970 Film Reference Guide for Medicine and Allied Health Sciences
    1969 Film Reference Guide for Medicine and Allied Sciences
    1967 Public Health Service Film Catalog
    Radiological Health Training Resources Catalog
    Selected Audiovisuals on Mental Health
    Selected List: Alcohol and Drug Problems
    Union List of Audiovisuals in the Library Network of the Veterans Administration
    Video Tape Catalog Continuing Medical Education and Instruction (AHSUSA)
    VA Film Catalog

QUACKERY

    Audiovisual Guide to the Catalog of Food and Drug Information and Educational Materials Center

RADIOLOGY
Radiation
X-Rays

    Army Films for Non-Profit Use
    Audiovisual Materials in Dental Auxiliary Education
    Cancer Film Guide
    Catalog of Films Available from Agencies: The U.S. Department of Commerce
    Dental Training Films
    Dentistry: A Select List of U.S. Government Produced Audiovisual Materials
    Energy Films Catalog
    Films: Free from the National Bureau of Standards
    Index of Army Motion Pictures for Public Non-Profit Use
    Medical Film Catalog
    NASA Film List
    National Library of Medicine Audiovisuals Catalog
    National Library of Medicine AVLINE Catalog
    National Medical Audiovisual Center Catalog: Films for the Health Sciences
    1970 Film Reference Guide for Medicine and Allied Health Sciences
    1969 Film Reference Guide for Medicine and Allied Sciences
    Radiological Health Training Resources Catalog
    Source Book of Educational Materials for Radiation Therapy
    Training Films [Mine Safety and Health Administration]
    Union List of Audiovisuals in the Library Network of the Veterans Administration
    VA Film Catalog

RAPE

    Media Resources Catalog
    Resources in Women's Educational Equity Non-Print Media and Materials

RELIGION

    Indians in the United States: Select Audiovisual Records
    Reference List of Audiovisual Materials Produced by the United States Government—Suppl., A
    Source Book of Educational Materials for Radiation Therapy
    VA Film Catalog

REPRODUCTION
    see **EVOLUTION (Humans and Primates)**

RESEARCH
    see also **EDUCATION, CONTINUING**

    Audio Visual Materials Catalog—Arthritis Information Clearinghouse
    Audiovisual Aids Directory of the Rehabilitational Research and Training Centers
    Audio-Visual Aids for High Blood Pressure Education
    Audiovisual Catalog of National Highway Traffic Safety Administration
    Catalog of Audio-Visual Aids in Hypertension
    Catalog of Training Films and Other Media for Special Education
    Criminal Justice Audiovisual Materials Directory
    Dental Training Films
    Directory of Cancer Research Information Resources
    Drug Abuse Films
    Drug Abuse Prevention Films: A Multicultural Film Catalog
    Energy Films Catalog
    Environmental Movies and Slide Shows from EPA
    FAA Film Catalog
    Federal Emergency Management Agency Motion Picture Catalog
    Film Archives on Child Development—The Inauguration of the Child Development Archives
    Film Catalog 1980. Pacific Region
    Film Guide on Reproduction and Development
    Index of Army Motion Pictures for Public Non-Profit Use
    List of Audiovisual Materials Produced by the U.S. Government in History, A
    Media Resources Catalog
    NASA Film List
    NIOSH—Films and Filmstrips on Occupational Safety and Health
    NOAA Motion Picture Films
    Publications, Radio, Films, Slides, Fact Sheets, T.V.
    Radiological Health Training Resources Catalog
    Recent Film Releases of the U.S. Department of Agriculture
    Reference List of Audiovisual Materials Produced by the U.S. Government, A
    Selected Films: Heart Disease, Cancer, and Stroke
    Space Benefits; NASA Films and Publications Describing Benefits of Space Technology
    Video Tape Catalog Continuing Medical Education and Instruction (AHSUSA)

Subject Index

RECREATION
see **PHYSICAL FITNESS** . . .

REHABILITATION
General

> Adult Group Leader Guide for the Use with Dial A-L-C-O-H-O-L and Jackson Junior High
> AoA Catalog of Films on Aging
> Audiovisual Aids Directory of the Rehabilitation Research and Training Centers
> Audio Visual Materials Catalog—Arthritis Information Clearinghouse
> Catalog of Educational Captioned Films for the Deaf
> Catalog of Training Films and Other Media for Special Education
> Criminal Justice Audiovisual Materials Directory
> Drug Abuse Films
> In Focus: Alcohol and Alcoholism Media
> List of Audiovisual Materials Produced by the U.S. Government for Drug Abuse Prevention, A
> Media Resources Catalog
> Medical Film Catalog
> Mental Retardation Film List
> Medical Catalog of Selected Audiovisual Materials Produced by the U.S. Government
> National Library of Medicine Audiovisuals Catalog
> National Library of Medicine AVLINE Catalog
> National Medical Audiovisual Center Catalog: Films for the Health Sciences
> 1970 Film Reference Guide for Medicine and Allied Health Sciences
> 1967 Public Health Service Film Catalog
> Reference List of Audiovisual Materials Produced by the U.S. Government, A
> Union List of Audiovisuals in the Library Network of the Veterans Administration
> VA Film Catalog

RESPIRATORY SYSTEM

> National Library of Medicine Audiovisuals Catalog
> National Library of Medicine AVLINE Catalog
> National Medical Audiovisual Center Catalog: Films for the Health Sciences
> Training Films [Mine Safety and Health Administration]
> Union List of Audiovisuals in the Library Network of the Veterans Administration
> VA Film Catalog

SAFETY
Accident Prevention Environmental Health
Occupational Safety
Protective Devises

> AoA Catalog of Films on Aging
> Army Films for Non-Profit Use
> Audiovisual Catalog of National Highway Traffic Safety Administration
> Bimonthly List of Publications and Audiovisuals
> Catalog of Educational Captioned Films for the Deaf
> Catalog of the United States Coast Guard Films
> Catalog of Films Available from Agencies: The U.S. Department of Commerce Serving the Nation

SAFETY (continued)

Directory of Cancer Research Information Resources
Disaster Preparedness: Publications, Films, and Other Audio-Visual Materials from the National Weather Service
Energy Films Catalog
Engineering: Selected U.S. Government Audiovisuals
FAA Film Catalog
Federal Emergency Management Agency Motion Picture Catalog
Films: Free from the National Bureau of Standards
Film Resources on Japan
Forest Service Films Available on Loan to the Public for Educational Purposes
Library of Congress Catalogs: Audiovisual Materials
List of Audiovisual Materials Produced by the U.S. Government for Consumer Education, A
List of Audiovisual Materials Produced by the U.S. Government for Emergency Medical Service, A
List of Audiovisual Materials Produced by the U.S. Government for Fire/Law Enforcement, A
List of Audiovisual Materials Produced by the U.S. Government for Flight and Meteorology, A
List of Audiovisual Materials Produced by the U.S. Government for Industrial Safety, A
Listing of Educational Materials for Use by Schools
Medical Film Catalog
NASA Film List
Natural Resources Department Films
NIOSH—Films and Filmstrips on Occupational Safety and Health
Publications, Radio, Films, Slides, Fact Sheets, T.V.
Quarterly Update: A Comprehensive Listing of New Audiovisual Materials and Services Offered by the National Audiovisual Center
Radiological Health Training Resources Catalog
Recent Film Releases of the U.S. Department of Agriculture
Reference List of Audiovisual Materials Produced by the U.S. Government, A
Reference List of Audiovisual Materials Produced by the United States Government, A
Resource File: Practical Publications for Energy Management. A Reference Guide to Handbooks, Curricula, and Audiovisual Materials, The
Training Film [Mine Safety and Health Administration]
VA Film Catalog

SANITATION

Audiovisual Guide to the Catalog of the Food and Nutrition Information and Educational Materials Center
Engineering: Selected U.S. Government Audiovisuals
Environmental Movies and Slide Shows from EPA
Guide to Audiovisual Aids for Spanish-Speaking Americans
Medical Film Catalog
VA Film Catalog

Subject Index

SCIENCE
General

Catalog of Educational Captioned Films for the Deaf
Catalog of Training Films and Other Media for Special Education
Educational Media Resources in Egypt
Federal Emergency Management Agency Motion Picture Catalog
Film Catalog
Film Fare: A Catalog of Films and Filmstrips Produced by the U.S. Department of Housing and Urban Development
Film: Free from the National Bureau of Standards
List of Educational Aids
Materials from the National Arts and the Handicapped Information Service: Annotated Bibliography
NOAA Motion Picture Films
Quarterly Update: A Comprehensive Listing of New Audiovisual Materials and Services Offered by the National Audiovisual Center
Recent Film Releases of the U.S. Department of Agriculture
Reference List of Audiovisual Materials Produced by the U.S. Government, A
Selected Educational Media
Smithsonian Slide Series: Slides. Filmstrips. Audiocassettes. Booklets.

SEX AND SEX EDUCATION
see also **FAMILY PLANNING**

Audiovisual Aids Directory of the Rehabilitation Research and Training Centers
Child Abuse and Neglect Audiovisual Materials
Film Archives on Child Development—The Inauguration of the Child Development Archives
Library of Congress Catalogs: Audiovisual Materials
Medical Catalog of Selected Audiovisual Materials Produced by the U.S. Government
National Library of Medicine Audiovisuals Catalog
National Library of Medicine AVLINE Catalog
National Medical Audiovisual Center Catalog: Films for the Health Sciences
1970 Film Reference Guide for Medicine and Allied Health Sciences
Resources in Women's Educational Equity Non-Profit Media and Materials
Selected Audiovisuals on Mental Health
Union List of Audiovisuals in the Library Network of the Veterans Administration
Venereal Disease Films for the General Public

SKIN
see **DERMATOLOGY**

SLEEP AND DREAMS
see also **PSYCHIATRY AND PSYCHOLOGY**

Union List of Audiovisual Materials in the Library Network of the Veterans Administration

SOCIAL SCIENCES

    AoA Catalog of Films on Aging
    Adult Group Leader Guide for the Use with Dial A-L-C-O-H-O-L and Jackson Junior High
    Audiovisual Aids Directory of the Rehabilitation Research and Training
    Catalog of Educational Captioned Films for the Deaf
    Catalog of Training Films and Other Media for Special Education
    Child Abuse and Neglect Audiovisual Materials
    Criminal Justice Audiovisual Materials Directory
    Documentary Film Classics Produced by the U.S. Government
    Drug Abuse Films
    Drug Abuse Prevention Films: A Multicultural Film Catalog
    Educational Media Resources in Egypt
    Film Resources on Japan
    Health
    Guide to Audio-Visual Aids for Courses in History of Latin American Civlization in Higher Education Institutions, A
    Guide to Audiovisual Aids for Spanish-Speaking Americans
    In Focus: Alcohol and Alcoholism Media
    List of Audiovisual Materials Produced by the U.S. Government for Social Sciences, A
    List of Audiovisual Materials Produced by the U.S. Government—Spanish Language Soundtracks, A
    Media Resources Catalog
    Medical Catalog of Selected Audiovisual Materials Produced by the U.S. Government
    Mental Retardation Film List
    National Library of Medicine Audiovisuals Catalog
    National Library of Medicine AVLINE Catalog
    National Medical Audiovisual Center Catalog: Films for the Health Sciences
    Quarterly Update: A Comprehensive Listing of New Audiovisual Materials and Services Offered by the National Audiovisual Center
    Reference List of Audiovisual Materials Produced by the U.S. Government, A
    Reference List of Audiovisual Materials Produced by the United States Government—Suppl., A
    Union List of Audiovisuals in the Library Network of the Veterans Administration
    Video Tape Catalog Continuing Medical Education and Instruction (AHSUSA)
    VA Film Catalog

SOCIETIES
  Clubs
  Organizations

    Bimonthly List of Publications and Audiovisuals
    Child Abuse and Neglect Audiovisual Materials
    FAA Film Catalog for Public Use
    Film Catalog
    Film Resources on Japan
    Health
    In Focus: Alcohol and Alcoholism Media
    Radiological Health Training Resources Catalog
    Recent Film Releases of the U.S. Department of Agriculture

Subject Index

SOCIETIES (continued)

Selected Films: Heart Disease, Cancer, and Stroke
Where the Drug Films Are: A Guide to Evaluation Services and Distributors

SPACE SCIENCES

Energy Films Catalog
Engineering: Selected U.S. Government Audiovisuals
Federal Emergency Management Agency Motion Picture Catalog
List of Audiovisual Materials Produced by the United States Government for Flight and Meteorology, A
Library of Congress Catalogs: Audiovisual Materials
List of Educational Aids
Medical Catalog of Selected Audiovisual Materials Produced by the U.S. Government
Medical Film Catalog
NASA Film List
NOAA Motion Picture Films
Reference List of Audiovisual Materials Produced by the U.S. Government, A
Reference List of Audiovisual Materials Produced by the United States Government—Suppl., A
Recent Film Releases of the U.S. Department of Agriculture
Selected Educational Media
Smithsonian Slide Series: Slides. Filmstrips. Audiocassettes. Booklets.
Space Benefits: NASA Films and Publications Describing Benefits of Space Technology
Viking Film Announcement

SPORTS
see **PHYSICAL FITNESS** ...

STATISTICS AND STANDARDS

Audiovisual Catalog of National Highway and Safety Administration
Catalog of Films Available from Agencies: The U.S. Department of Commerce Serving the Nation
Films: Free from the National Bureau of Standards
Environmental Movies and Slide Shows from EPA
Recent Film Releases of the U.S. Department of Agriculture
Source Book of Educational Materials for Radiation Therapy
Training Films [Mine Safety and Health Administration]

SUBMARINE MEDICINE
see **MARINE SCIENCES**

SURGERY

Army Films for Non-Profit Use
Audiovisual Materials in Dental Auxiliary Education
Audiovisual Aids Directory of the Rehabilitation Research and Training Centers
Cancer Film Guide
Dentistry: A Select List of U.S. Government Produced Audiovisual Materials
Dental Training Films

SURGERY (continued)

 Library of Congress Catalogs: Audiovisual Materials
 List of Educational Aids
 Medical Catalog of Selected Audiovisual Materials Produced by the U.S. Government
 Medical Film Catalog
 National Library of Medicine Audiovisuals Catalog
 National Library of Medicine AVLINE Catalog
 National Medical Audiovisual Center Catalog: Films for the Health Sciences
 1970 Film Reference Guide for Medicine and Allied Health Sciences
 1969 Film Reference Guide for Medicine and Allied Sciences
 1967 Public Health Service Film Catalog
 Reference List of Audiovisual Materials Produced by the U.S. Government, A
 Union List of Audiovisuals in the Library Network of the Veterans Administration
 Video Tape Catalog Continuing Medical Education and Instruction (AHSUSA)
 VA Film Catalog

SURGERY, PLASTIC

 Cancer Film Guide
 Criminal Justice Audiovisual Materials Directory
 Dental Training Films
 Dentistry: A Select List of U.S. Government Produced Audiovisual Materials
 Library of Congress Catalogs: Audiovisual Materials
 Medical Catalog of Selected Audiovisuals Produced by the U.S. Government
 Medical Film Catalog
 1970 Film Reference Guide for Medicine and Allied Health Sciences
 1969 Film Reference Guide for Medicine and Allied Sciences
 1967 Public Health Service Film Catalog
 Union List of Audiovisuals in the Library Network of the Veterans Administration
 VA Film Catalog
 Video Tape Catalog Continuing Medical Education and Instruction (AHSUSA)

TECHNOLOGY
General

 Audiovisual Guide to the Catalog for the Food and Nutrition Information and Educational Materials Center
 Catalog of the United States Coast Guard Films
 Dental Training Films
 Educational Media Resources on Egypt
 Energy Efficiency Sharing: Business-to-Business Program to Facilitate Exchange of Energy Management Technology and Techniques
 Energy Films Catalog
 Films: Free fom the National Bureau of Standards
 Guide to Audio-Visual Aids for Courses in the History of Latin American Civilization in Higher Education Institutions, A
 Library of Congress Catalogs: Audiovisual Materials
 List of Educational Aids
 Medical Catalog of Selected Audiovisual Materials Produced by the U.S. Government
 Medical Film Catalog
 NASA Film List
 National Library of Medicine Audiovisuals Catalog

Subject Index

TECHNOLOGY (continued)

National Library of Medicine AVLINE Catalog
National Medical Audiovisual Center Catalog: Films for the Health Sciences
NOAA Motion Picture Films
Problems in Bibliographic Access to Non-Print Materials: a Report
Publications, Radio, Films, Slides, Fact Sheets, T.V.
Recent Film Releases of the U.S. Department of Agriculture
Smithsonian Slide Series: Slides. Filmstrips. Audiocassettes. Booklets.
Source Book of Educational Materials for Radiation Therapy
Space Benefits: NASA Films and Publications Describing Benefits of Space Technology
Training Films [Mine Safety and Health Administration]
Union List of Audiovisuals in the Library Network of the Veterans Administration

TISSUE CULTURE
see CYTOLOGY . . .

THANATOLOGY

Audiovisual Aids Directory of the Rehabilitation Research and Training Centers
Audiovisual Catalog of National Highway Traffic Safety Administration
Educational Media Resources in Egypt
List of Audiovisual Materials Produced by the U.S. Government for Consumer Education, A
NASA Film List
National Library of Medicine Audiovisuals Catalog
National Library of Medicine AVLINE Catalog
National Medical Audiovisual Center Catalog: Films for the Health Sciences
Selected Audiovisuals on Mental Health
Source Book of Educational Materials for Radiation Therapy
Union List of Audiovisuals in the Library Network of the Veterans Administration
VA Film Catalog

TOMOGRAPHY

Source Book of Educational Materials for Radiation Therapy

TOXICOLOGY
Poisons
see also CHEMISTRY . . .
    POISONING

List of Audiovisual Materials Produced by the U.S. Government for Flight and Meteorology, A
List of Educational Aids
NASA Film List
National Library of Medicine Audiovisuals Catalog
National Library of Medicine AVLINE Catalog
National Medical Audiovisual Center Catalog: Films for the Health Sciences
1970 Film Reference Guide for Medicine and Allied Health Sciences
1969 Film Reference Guide for Medicine and Allied Sciences
1967 Public Health Service Film Catalog

Subject Index

TOXICOLOGY (continued)

    Publications, Radio, Films, Slides, Fact Sheets, T.V.
    Reference List of Audiovisual Materials Produced by the U.S. Government, A
    Union List of Audiovisuals in the Library Network of the Veterans Administration

TOXINS
    see **CHEMISTRY** ...
        POISONING
        TOXICOLOGY

TRANSPORTATION
    Air
    Land
    Sea

        Audiovisual Catalog of the National Highway Traffic and Safety Administration
        Educational Media Resource on Egypt
        Environmental Movies and Slide Shows from EPA
        FAA Film Catalog for Public Use
        Film Fare: A Catalog of Films and Filmstrips Produced by the U.S. Department of House and Urban Development
        Film Resources in Japan
        List of Audiovisual Materials Produced by the U.S. Government for Industrial Safety, A
        Reference List of Audiovisual Materials Produced by the U.S. Government, A
        Smithsonian Slide Series. Slides. Filmstrips. Audiocassettes. Booklets.
        Space Benefits: NASA Films and Publications Describing Benefits of Space Technology
        35 Energy Films
        Resource File: Practical Publications for Energy Management. A Reference Guide to Handbooks, Curricula, and Audiovisual Materials, The
        Training Films [Mine Safety and Health Administration]

TROPICAL MEDICINE

    Index to Army Motion Pictures for Public Non-Profit Use
    Medical Film Catalog

URBAN HEALTH
    City Planning
    see also **COMMUNITY HEALTH**
        PUBLIC HEALTH

        Adult Group Leader Guide for the Use with Dial A-L-C-O-H-O-L and Jackson Junior High
        Catalog of Training Films and Other Media for Special Education
        Film Fare: A Catalog of Films and Filmstrips Produced by the U.S. Department of Housing and Urban Development
        Film Resources on Japan
        Guide to Audio-Visual Aids for Courses in the History of Latin American Civilization in Higher Education Institutions, A

Subject Index

URBAN HEALTH (continued)

    List of Audiovisual Materials Produced by the U.S. Government for Consumer Education, A
    Medical Catalog of Selected Audiovisual Materials Produced by the U.S. Government
    Selected Educational Media

UROGENITAL SYSTEM

    Audiovisual Aids Directory of the Rehabilitation Research and Training Centers
    National Library of Medicine Audiovisuals Catalog
    National Library of Medicine AVLINE Catalog
    National Medical Audiovisual Center Catalog: Films for the Health Sciences
    1970 Film Reference Guide for Medicine and Allied Health Sciences
    Union List of Audiovisuals in the Library Network of the Veterans Administration

VETERINARY MEDICINE
  see also **ZOOLOGY**

    Catalog of Films Available from Agencies: The U.S. Department of Commerce Serving the Nation
    Library of Congress Catalogs: Audiovisual Materials
    List of Educational Aids
    Medical Film Catalog
    National Library of Medicine AVLINE Catalog
    1970 Film Reference Guide for Medicine and Allied Health Sciences
    1969 Film Reference Guide for Medicine and Allied Sciences
    1967 Public Health Service Films Catalog
    Union List of Audiovisuals in the Library Network of the Veterans Administration
    Video Tape Catalog Continuing Medical Education and Instruction (AHSUSA)

VOCATIONAL GUIDANCE
  see **CAREERS**

VOCATIONAL TRAINING
  see **CAREERS**

VOLUNTARY HEALTH AGENCIES

    Audio Visual Materials Catalog—Arthritis Information Clearinghouse
    Child Abuse and Neglect Audiovisual Materials
    List of Audiovisual Materials Produced by the U.S. Government for Foreign Language Instruction, A
    Union List of Audiovisuals in the Library Network of the Veterans Administration

WAR
  see also **DISASTERS**
        HOSPITALS OVERSEAS . . . (Miscellaneous)

    Army Films for Non-Profit Use
    Documentary Film Classics Produced by the U.S. Government
    Index of Army Motion Pictures for Public Non-Profit Use

Subject Index

WAR (continued)

    Indians in the United States: Selected Audiovisual Records
    List of Audiovisual Materials Produced by the U.S. Government in History, A

WEATHER
    see CLIMATE

WILDLIFE
    see also ZOOLOGY

    Bimonthly List of Publications and Audiovisuals
    Educational Media Resources in Egypt
    Environmental Movies and Slide Shows from EPA
    Film Catalog
    Film Catalog 1980. Pacific Northern Region
    Film Resources on Japan
    Forest Service Films Available on Loan to the Public for Educational Pruposes
    Indians in the United States: Select Audiovisual Records
    Recent Film Releases of the U.S. Department of Agriculture

WOMEN
    see MEN AND WOMEN

WORLD HEALTH

    Audiovisual Catalog of the National Highway Traffic Safety Administration
    Audiovisual Guide to the Catalog of the Food and Nutrition Information and Educational Materials Center
    Catalog of Training Films and Other Media for Special Education
    Directory of Cancer Research Information Resources
    Documentary Film Classics Produced by the U.S. Government
    Educational Media Resources on Egypt
    Engineering: Selected U.S. Government Audiovisuals
    FAA Film Catalog for Public Use
    Film Resources in Japan
    Guide to Audio-Visual Aids for Courses in History of Latin American Civilization in Higher Education Institutions, A
    Index of Army Motion Pictures for Public Non-Profit Use
    Library of Congress Catalogs: Audiovisual Materials
    List of Audiovisual Materials Produced by the U.S. Government in History, A
    List of Audiovisual Materials Produced by the U.S. Government for Foreign Language Instruction, A
    Medical Film Catalog
    NASA Film List
    National Library of Medicine Audiovisuals Catalog
    National Library of Medicine AVLINE Catalog
    National Medical Audiovisual Center Catalog: Films for the Health Sciences
    1970 Film Reference Guide for Medicine and Allied Health Sciences
    1967 Public Health Service Film Catalog
    NOAA Motion Picture Films
    Radiological Health Training Resources Catalog
    Recent Film Releases of the U.S. Department of Agriculture

Subject Index

WORLD HEALTH (continued)

    Space Benefits: NASA Films and Publications Describing Benefits of Space and Technology
    Smithsonian Slide Series: Slides. Filmstrips. Audiocassettes. Booklets.

X-RAYS
    see **RADIOLOGY**

YOGA
    see also **PHYSICAL FITNESS**

    Union List of Audiovisual Materials in the Library Network of the Veterans Administration

ZOOLOGY
    see also **ENVIRONMENTAL SCIENCES**
        EVOLUTION
        VETERINARY MEDICINE
        WILDLIFE

    Bimonthly List of Publications and Audiovisuals
    Catalog of Educational Captioned Films for the Deaf
    Catalog of Films Available from Agencies: The U.S. Department of Commerce Serving the Nation
    Film Archives on Child Development—The Inauguration of the Child Development Archives
    Film Catalog
    Library of Congress Catalogs: Audiovisual Materials
    Film Catalog 1980. Pacific Northern Region
    National Library of Medicine Audiovisuals Catalog
    National Library of Medicine AVLINE Catalog
    National Medical Audiovisual Center Catalog: Films for the Health Sciences
    1970 Film Reference Guide for Medicine and Allied Health Sciences
    Recent Film Releases of the U.S. Department of Agriculture
    Selected Audiovisuals on Mental Health
    Selected Guide to Audio-Visual Materials on Alcohol and Alcoholism, A
    Smithsonian Slide Series: Slides. Filmstrips. Audiocassettes. Booklets.